# REMOVALS

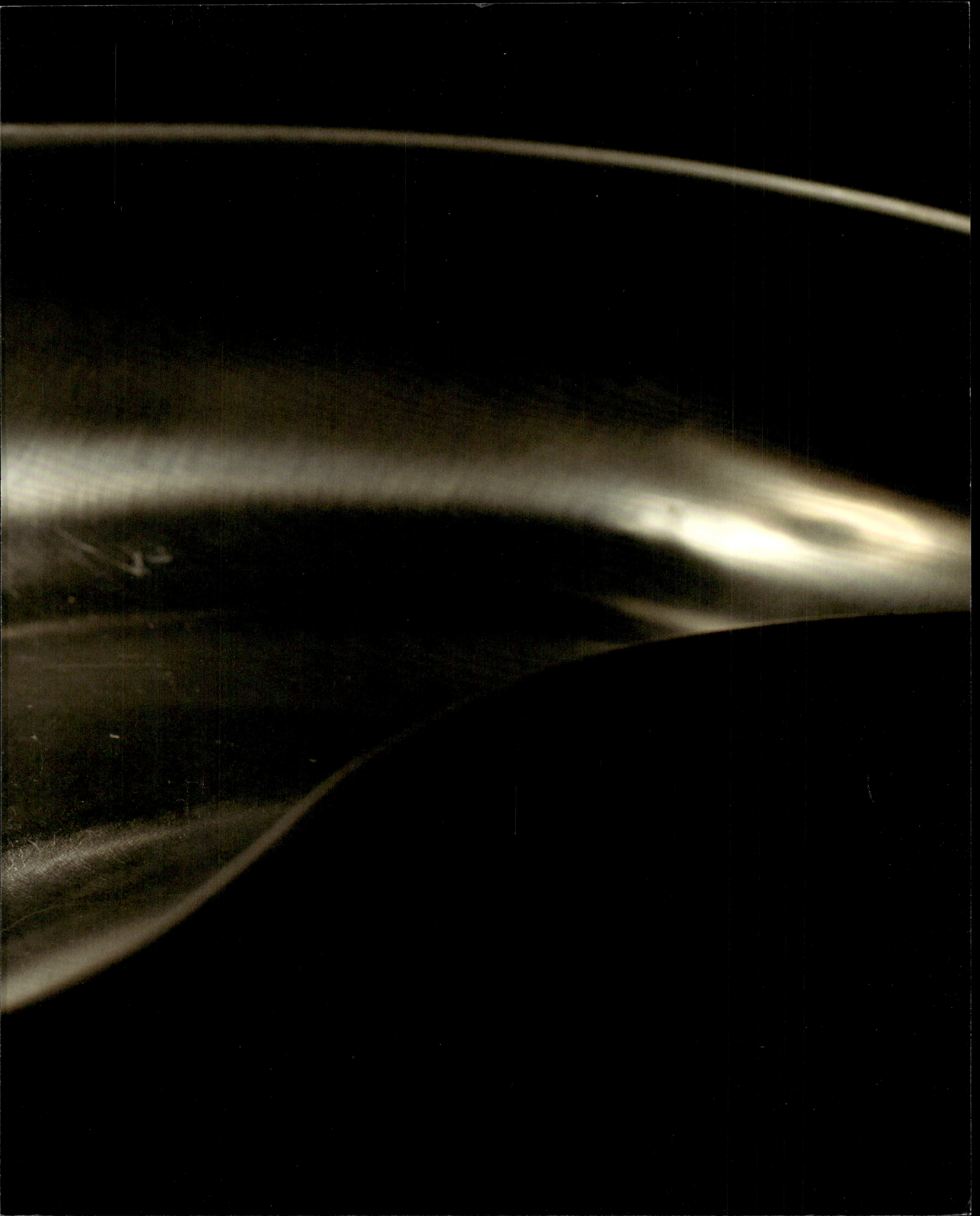

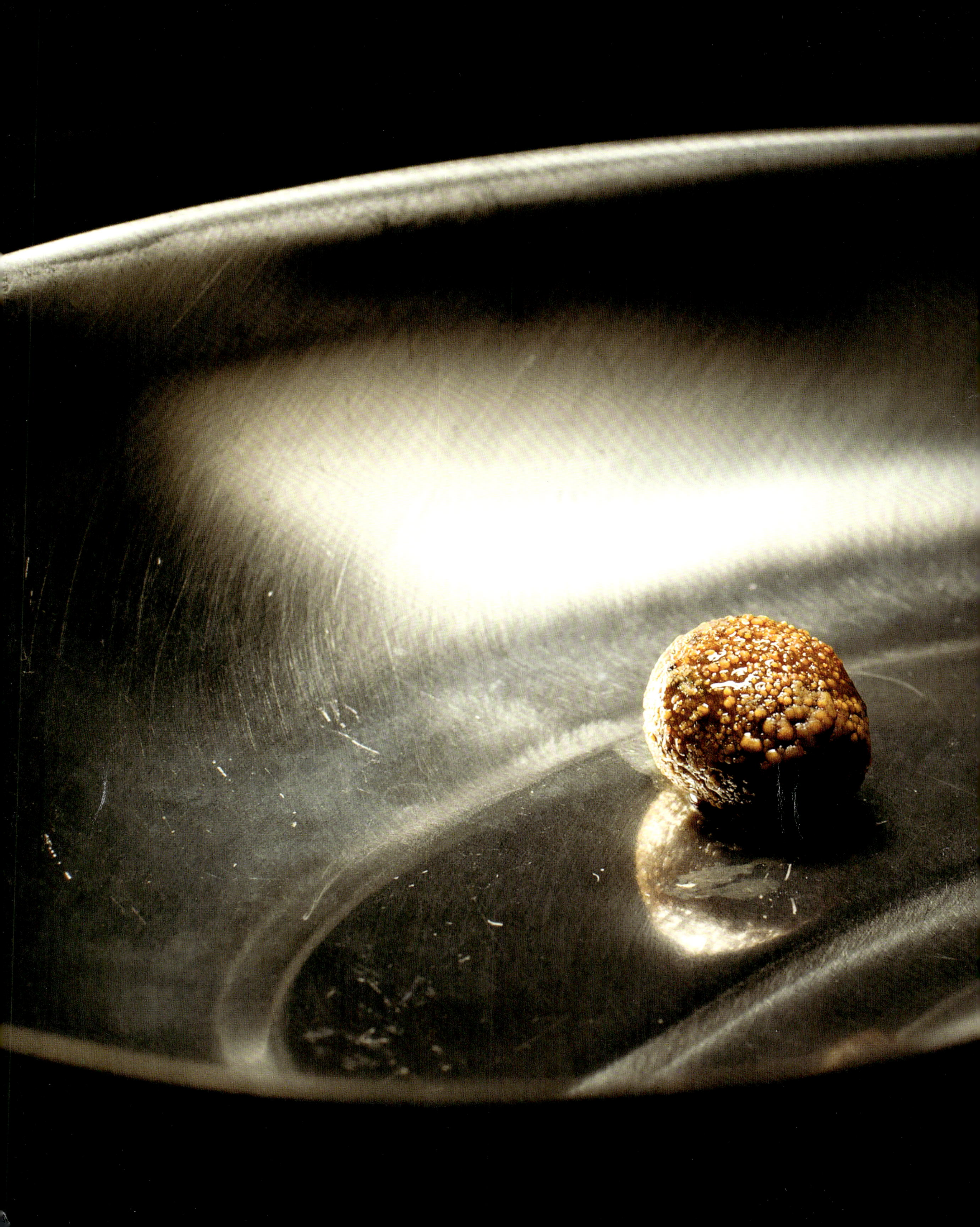

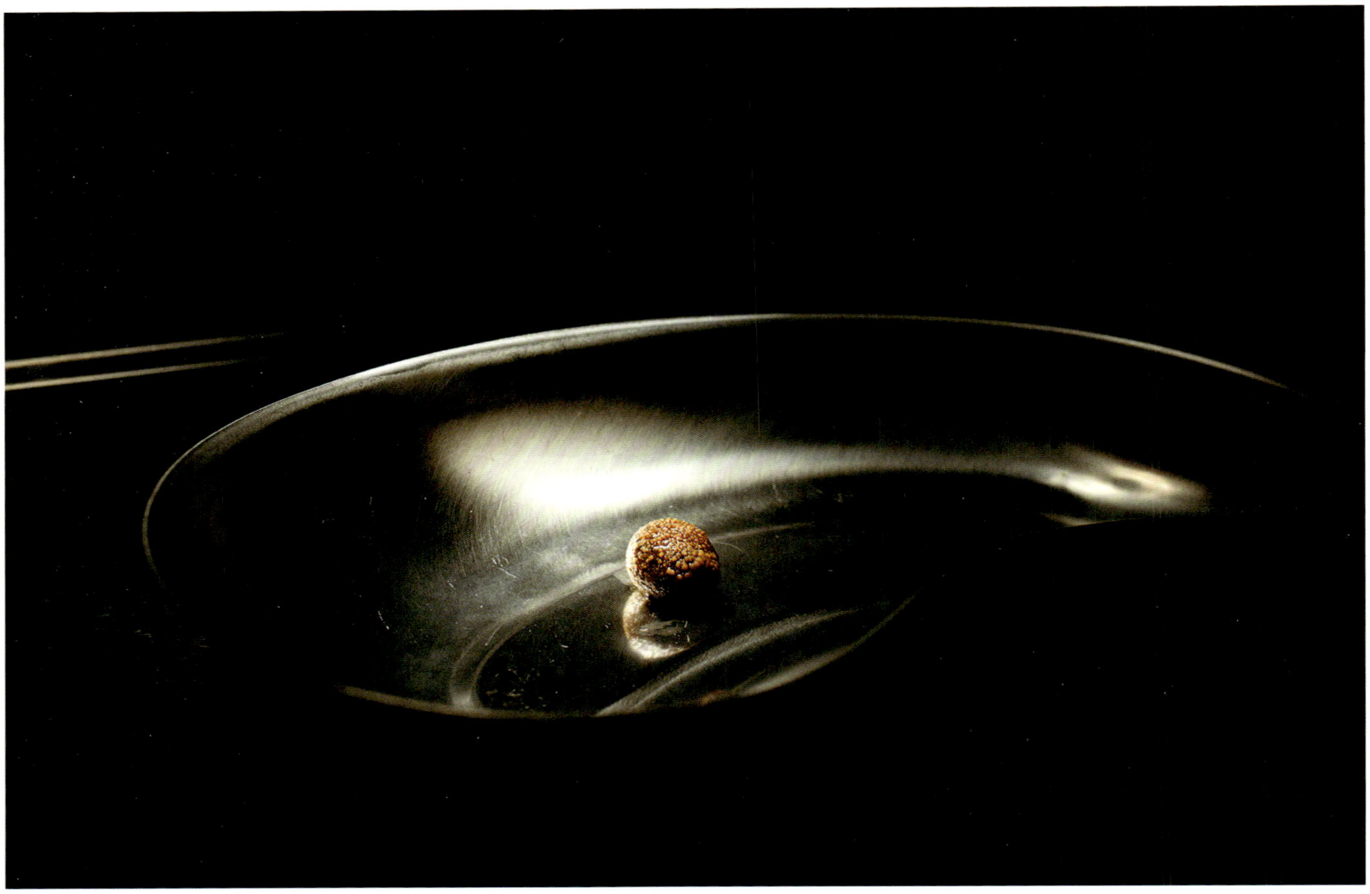

| SURGEON B | SURGEON A | SURGEON M |
| --- | --- | --- |
| *So, a fat-female-fifty. A cholesterol stone.* | *It's funny that there's just one stone. I can't remember many cases of gallstones with only one lump. Usually it's full of lumps, kind of like a cobblestone street. Personally, I at least like it in gallstone surgeries when you can cut it open, and they're so nicely interlaced, like a small mosaic of gallstones.* | *Cobblestones.* |
| | *Yeah.* | |
| *Do you think, if that one is dropped into the bowl, it goes 'plink' or 'plop'? It's got to be 'plink'.* | *That one must be...* | *That's probably pretty hard.* |
| | *But they're often just like compartments, interlocking together, they're soft, green, or then they're this kind of firmer bile, and the color is gross and they smell pretty bad.* | *Aren't those ones a little bit yellow inside?* |
| *Yeah.* | *Yeah, at least with the little experience that I have with those. B had a lcc (laparoscopic cholecystechtomy) today.* | |
| *Yeah, it was a fat-female-forty and there was one three-millimeter stone, one that broke when I handled it. It was the very soft kind. Most likely she has had more of them and they must have gone through.* | | |

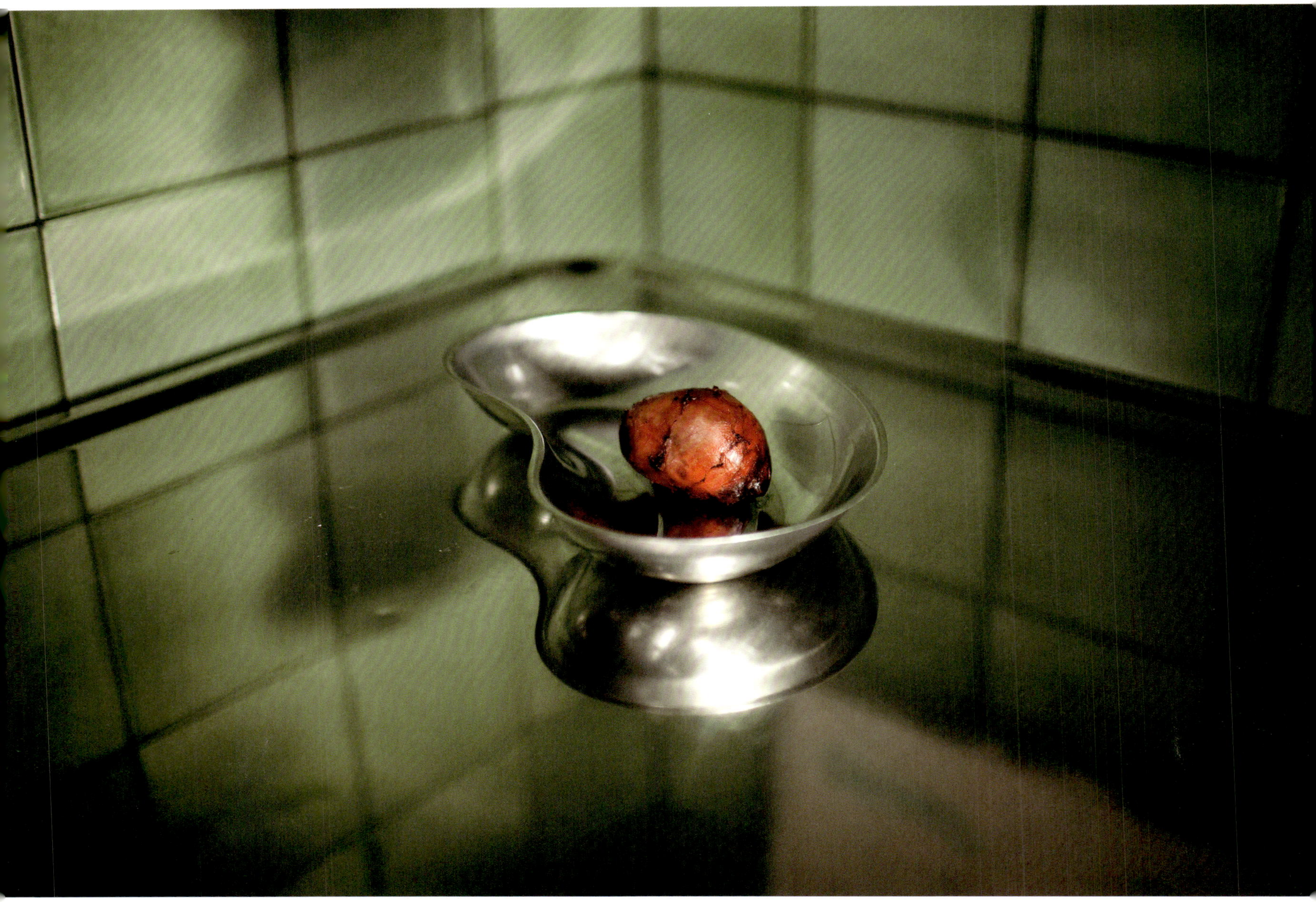

| SURGEON B | SURGEON A | SURGEON M |
|---|---|---|
| *What's that?* | *I could imagine that it's an umm…* | *Is it a goiter?* |
| | *Yeah, a goiter because they've probably used Harmonic and you can see the polar burn marks in lines right there. I could imagine it's a goiter.* | |
| *This is beautiful.* | *Yes it is, extremely beautiful.* | |
| *It must have caused symptoms.* | *That one must create some pressure. I guess the indication is right, if there's like half of an apple growing out of the neck.* | |
| *Yeah.* | *It's pretty big too.* | *It looks benign, there are no lumps, and the capsule looks intact.* |
| | *We are quite satisfied with this, aren't we?* | |

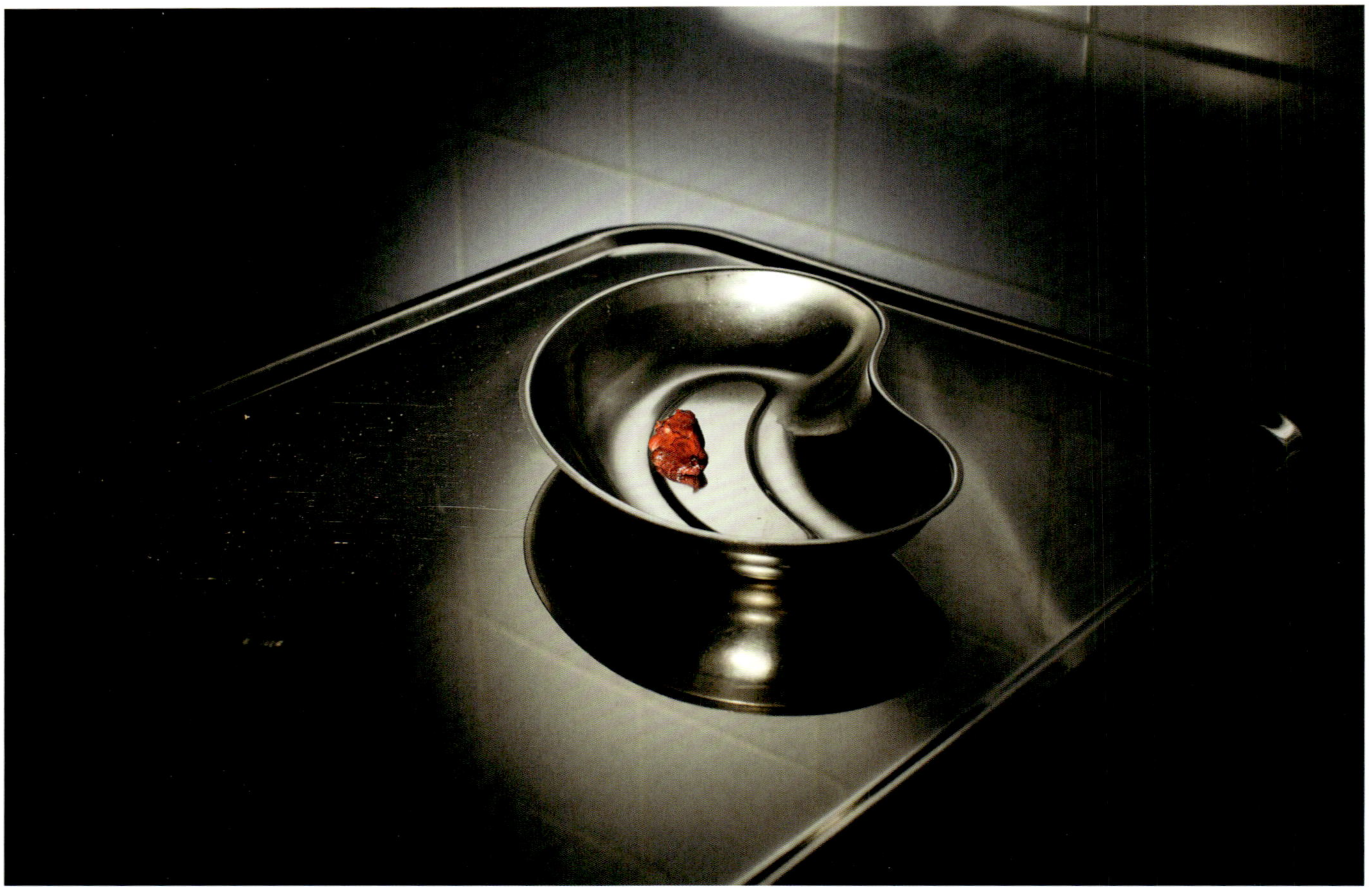

| SURGEON B | SURGEON A | SURGEON M |
| --- | --- | --- |
| *Is that a thyroid...* | *I don't know, it's some weird nodule anyway.* | |
| *Some cancer or something.* | | *That's lumpy at least.* |
| *Could it be thyroid...* | *Could it be something, some kind of lump anyway, with beautiful veins running on the surface.* | *Yeah, well it isn't a big lump, but even a small lump can cause a serious disease.*<br><br>*Have they removed the whole thyroid or a part of it?* |
| | *I could imagine that this is like, a half.* | |
| *Yeah.* | *Maybe it would be a bit larger, if it would be the whole.* | *Just a half of it then.* |
| | *Yeah.* | |

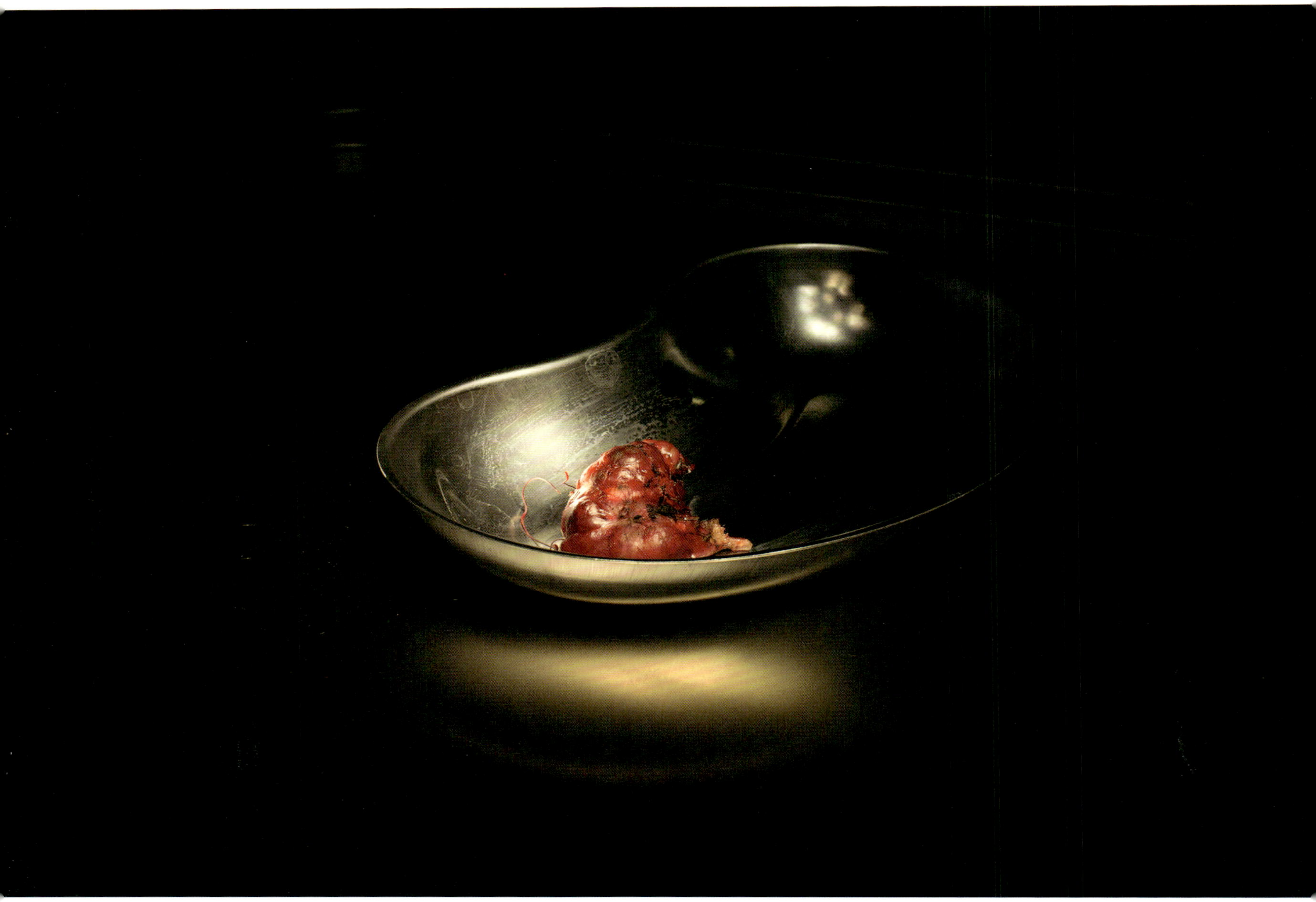

| SURGEON B | SURGEON A | SURGEON M |
|---|---|---|
| | *Well, this one looks like, at first glance it looks like some baby rat.* | *Yeah, like a rat fetus.* |
| | *Maybe a thyroid. A little bit sausage-like.* | *But it is also like...* |
| *Like cobblestones.* | | *Yes, it is nodular or something, like, there is no single cyst or growth of disease.* |
| | *Are these thyroid nodules, these lumps here?* | *So, if that's benign?*<br><br>*Still here the capsule looks relatively intact.* |
| | *There's a funny tail, a strip of some tissue over there. That's probably why it looks like the fetus of some mammal.* | *And then those clips there placed on the arteries.* |
| | *It looks like a nose.* | *Yes it does a little.* |

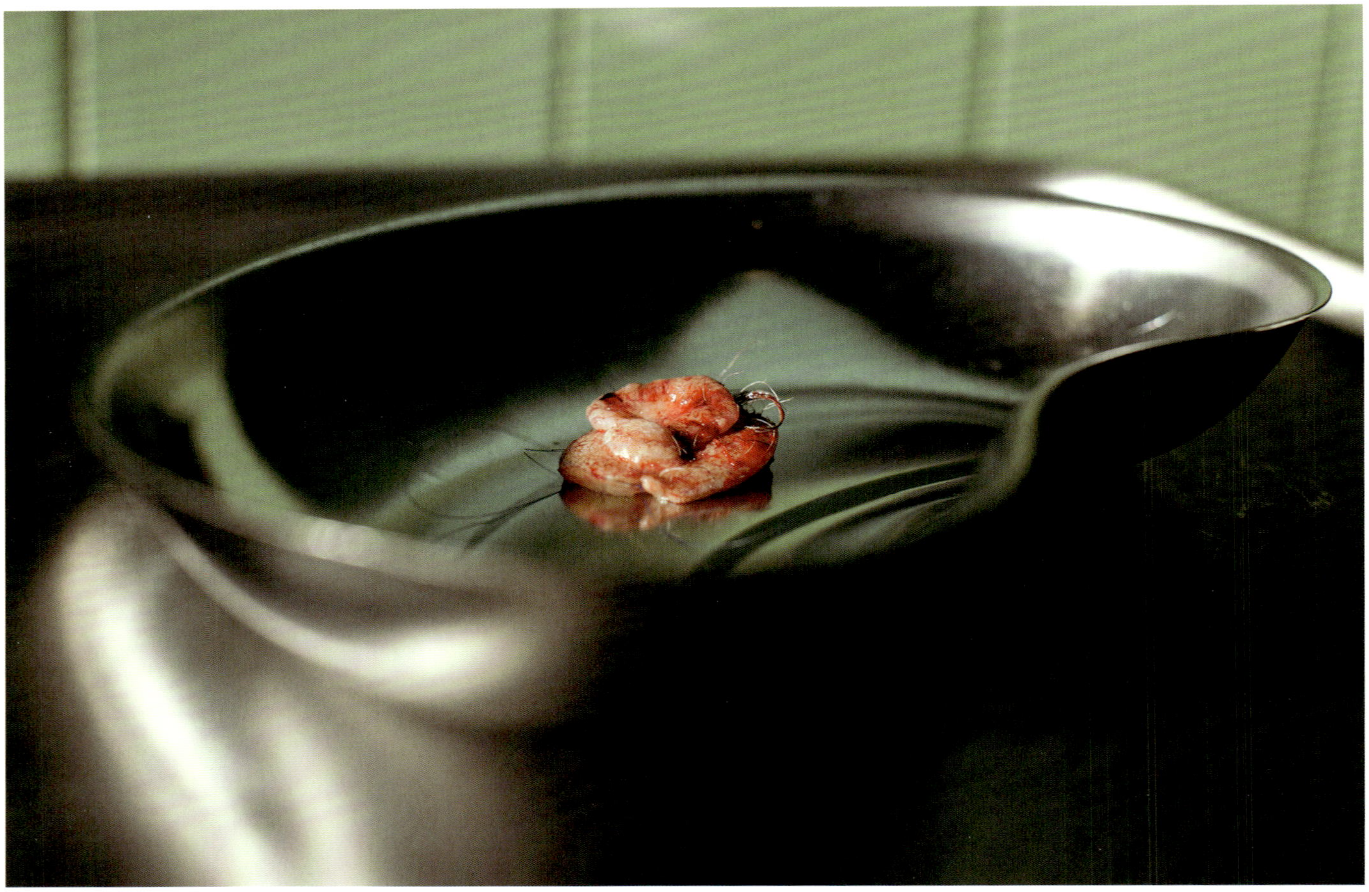

| SURGEON B | SURGEON A | SURGEON M |
| --- | --- | --- |
| *There's some kind of hair there. This is a teratoma. No, no it can't be a teratoma.* | *Or is it some skin tumor, isn't there skin there below?* | |
| *A little crater-like.* | *Is this some, like a basal-cell carcinoma anyway, or something similar. There's skin and hair.* | |
| *But then it would be removed with quite small margins.* | *I don't know, it does contract. If that's one of those with a stem...* | |
| *Okay.* | *...where the base is smaller in a way.* | |
| *So yeah, it is a basal-cell carcinoma.* | | *But is that supposed to be skin then?* |
| | *Doesn't that look like normal skin to you?* | |
| *At least there's hair.* | | *Yes.* |
| | *Could it be from the top of the head or from a temple or somewhere. Or if the other side has hair and that part doesn't. But it's true, the margins look rather small.* | *What's that lump on the left then?* |
| *Is that normal skin...* | | *No.* |
| *...in all its thickness there and here's the crater-like tumor and there's a little hair. Maybe it is removed from an area like the head, for example.* | *I could imagine it's on someone's temple. So there's skin there that's plate-like and growing.* | *Expanding from here to there and like...* |
| | *Yes, and going like this. (shows)* | *Yeah.* |
| *It's surprising that he didn't see the doctor earlier, if this has indeed been on the head.* | *Head with horns.* | *Indeed.* |

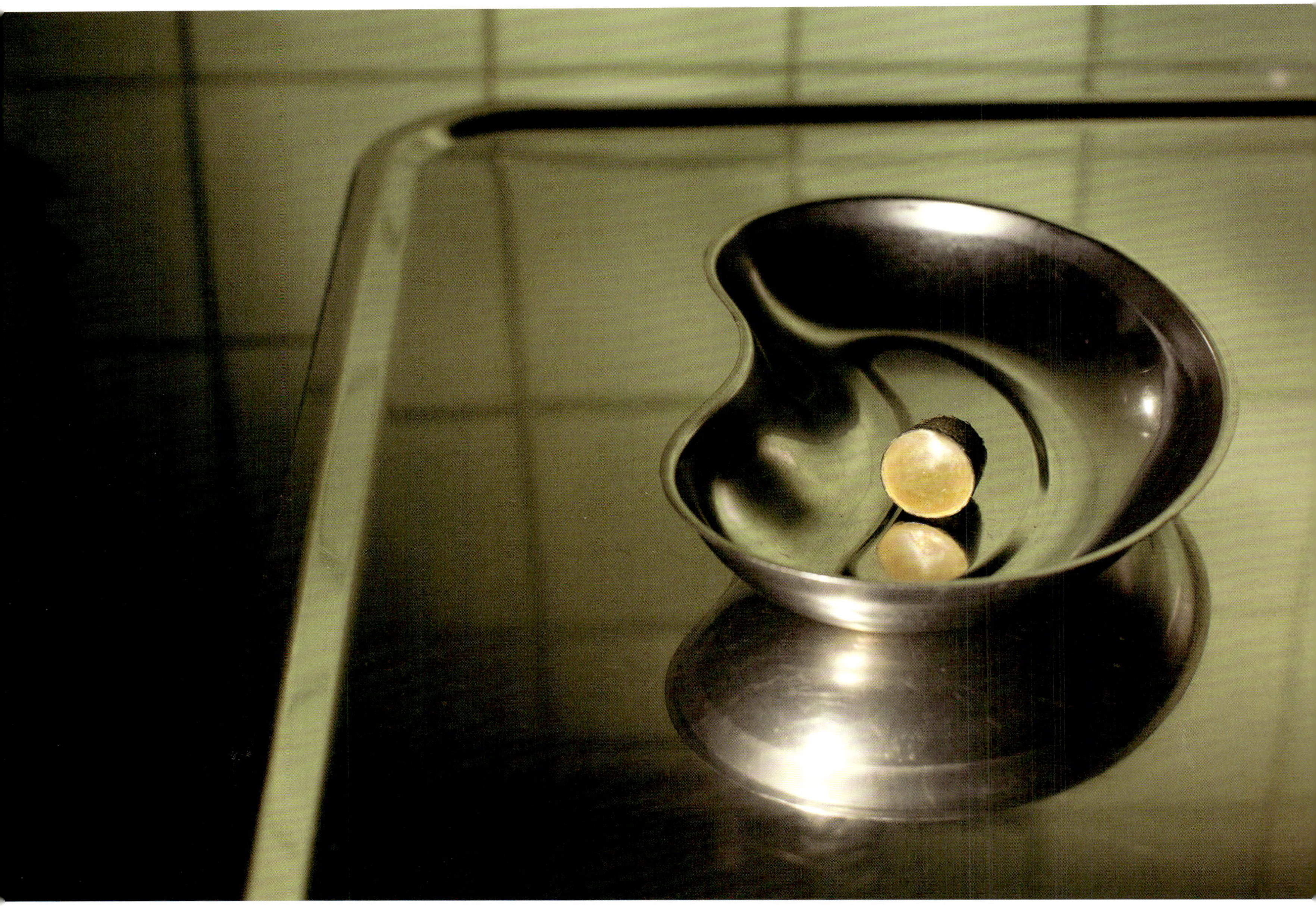

| SURGEON B | SURGEON A | SURGEON M |
| --- | --- | --- |
| *Is this a foreign body? No, what is this? The dark rim is quite even here. Could it be a split stone?* | *I don't know.* | *Quite black.* |
| | *Very black.* | *If I would see that one in a completely different context, I would think it's some chocolate truffle or the like.* |
| | *It does look like, it looks like one of those capsules you put in a coffee maker.* | |
| *No it's not a kidney stone. It is extremely large.* | *But aren't gallstones sometimes, like, completely black?* | |
| *They can be and then they can have different colors on the inside.* | | *But how were they able to slice it so clean?* |
| | *Yeah, it must be a stone.* | |
| *Gallstone. A nice one.* | *It's a capsule for a lavazza.* | |
| *It'll cause a fistula in the small intestine and also an ileus when it goes through.* | *Yes, it will.* | *That one won't go through.* |
| *I mean, if it goes through the opening of the fistula.* | | *Yes, yes.* |
| | *Then it causes contractions and you'll get a gallstone occlusion.* | |

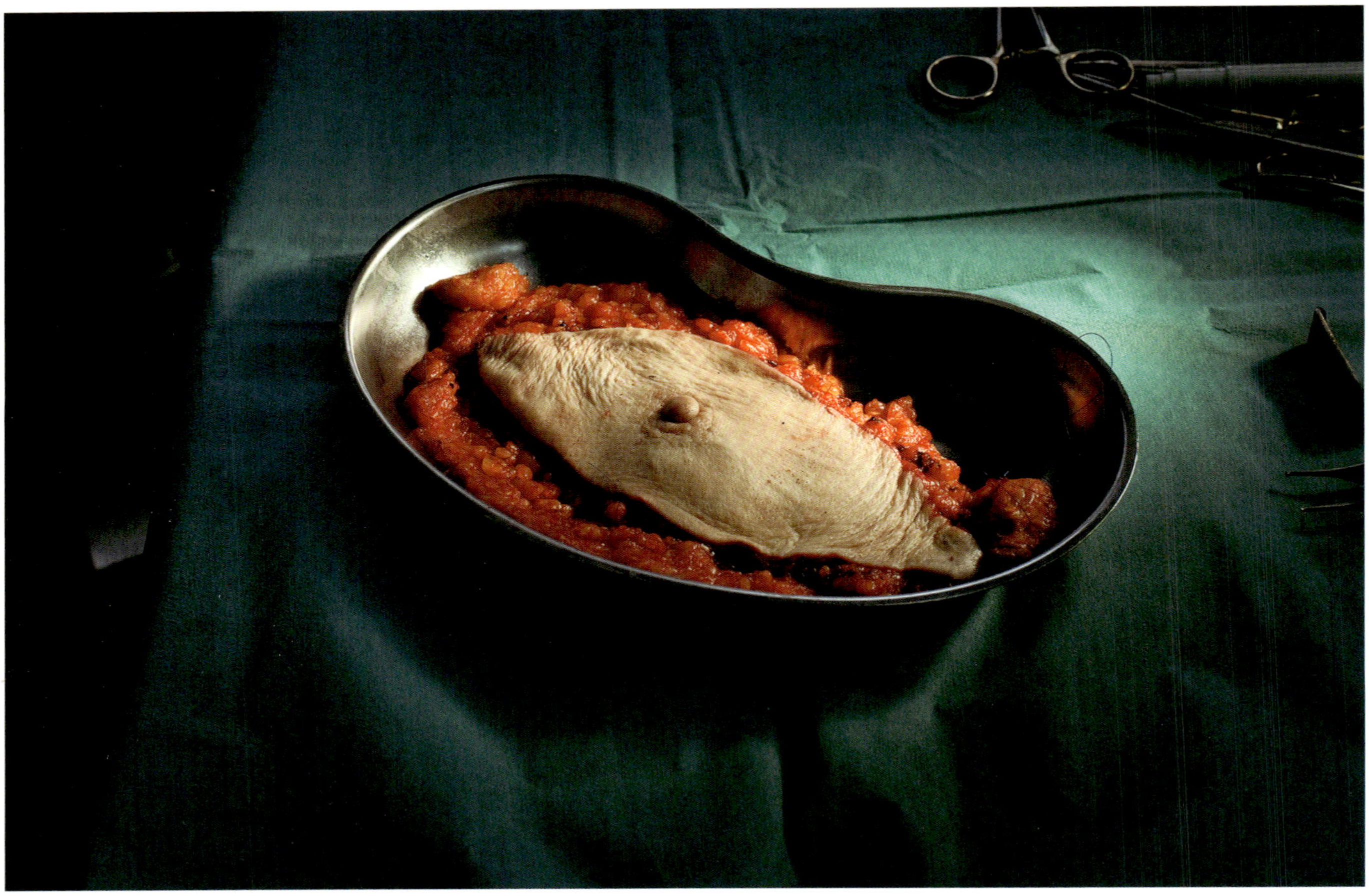

| SURGEON B | SURGEON A | SURGEON M |
|---|---|---|
| *That's a foot.* | *(laughs)* | *(laughs)* |
| | *A foot with a nipple.* | |
| *Yeah, don't you think? It's the big toe.* | | *This one isn't flatfooted but this one is...* |
| | *(laughs) A very bad ptosis of the breasts if the nipples are there in the feet. Yes, a breast.* | *Yeah, it's the whole breast?* |
| | *Yeah, this is a mastectomy all right.* | *A removal of the whole breast.* |
| | *Funny how symmetrical that piece of skin appears to be, because it isn't actually completely marquise shaped, is it. But it looks funny, kind of like an oval...* | *It's receded there.* |
| | *In fact it looks like an island in a sea of lava.* | |
| *(laughs)* | *If you just think about what it looks like aesthetically, without thinking about what it is.* | |
| *Yeah.* | *Or in some kind of lentil stew.* | |
| *Covered by ash.* | *An island covered in ash. Yes indeed.* | |
| *In lava.* | | *Are those lumps here mammary gland, the tumor must be somewhere in there...* |
| | *Yes, it's somewhere in there.* | *...hidden.* |
| *Medial. Is this the lateral side where the sutures are?* | *It always depends on which way you want to place it. I guess there's no systematic way. As long as you just place it on either side and remember where it is.* | |
| *I just meant that there's a sort of tail, so you could imagine that they have done an axillary evacuation.* | *Yes, maybe this is lateral after all.* | |

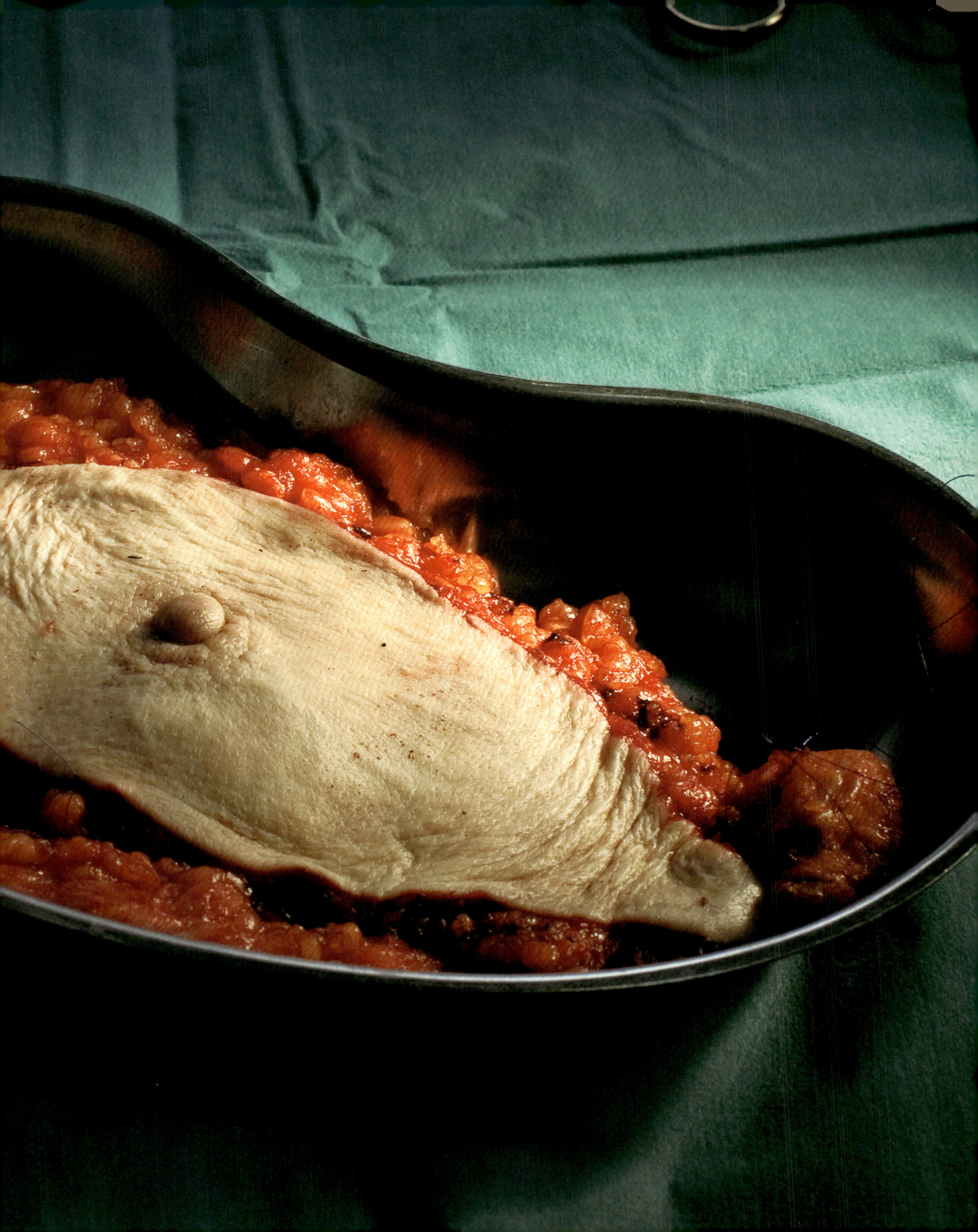

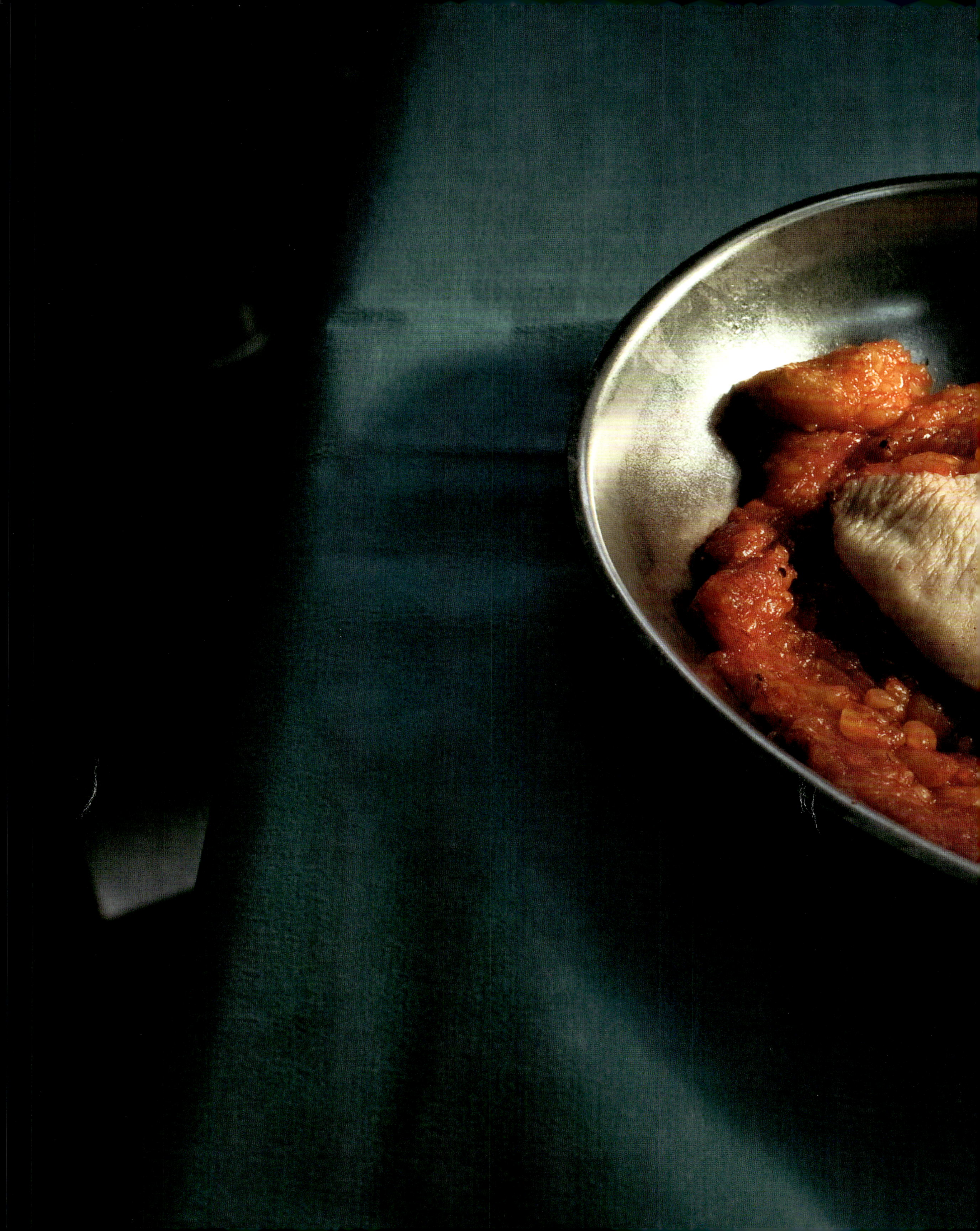

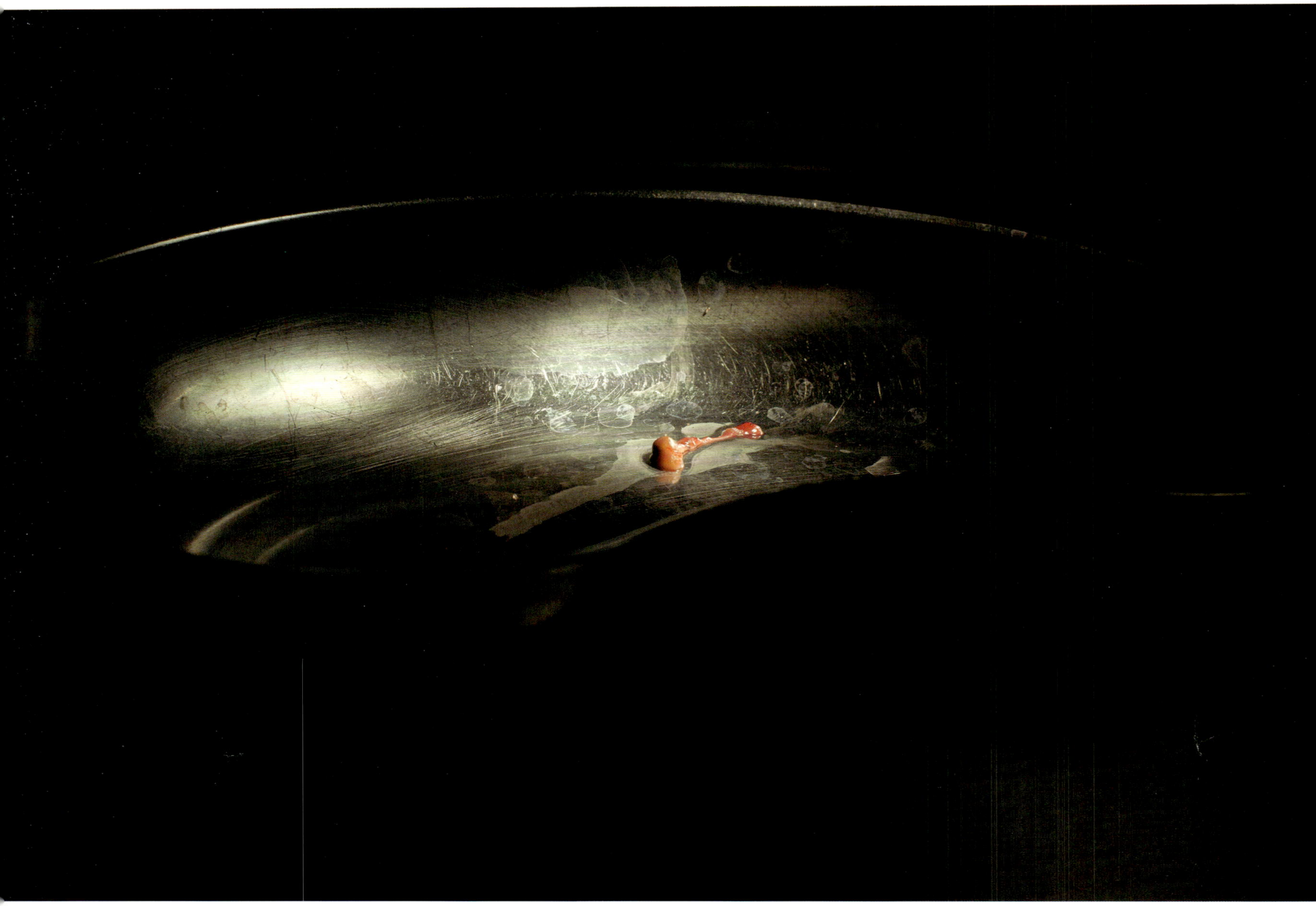

| SURGEON B | SURGEON A | SURGEON M |
|---|---|---|
| | | *Well, well...* |
| | *That's at least fat and some vein.* | |
| *Is it a biopsy?* | *A vein.*<br><br>*It could be a temporal arteritis biopsy, but one wouldn't put it in an emesis basin for God's sake.* | |
| *Or take that much fat to go.* | *And a man's forehead wouldn't have that much forehead-fat.* | |
| *No, there's almost no forehead-fat. (laughs)* | | |
| *I guess that's not it.* | *Well, there's some vein there anyway.* | |
| *Yeah.* | | *Well, well.* |
| | *Ectopic testis. Well look at that. An extra testis, and look, there's its wirings.* | *That testis has atrophied?* |
| *Where has it been?* | *It must have been there, up on the forehead.* | |
| | *(laughter)* | |
| | | *Has it been somewhere...* |
| | *Yeah, maybe in the scrotum or in the abdominal cavity, I don't know.* | *I don't know either.* |
| | *Seems strange...* | |
| *So this person then is, like, missing the other normal one?* | *Or could it be...* | |
| *An extra one.* | *...like, an extra one. I think this might be an extra one.* | *Yeah, I don't know. You can't suddenly have an extra one, can you?* |
| *It isn't a teratoma anyway, that little fella.* | *I guess not. It's a bit exceptional this one.* | |

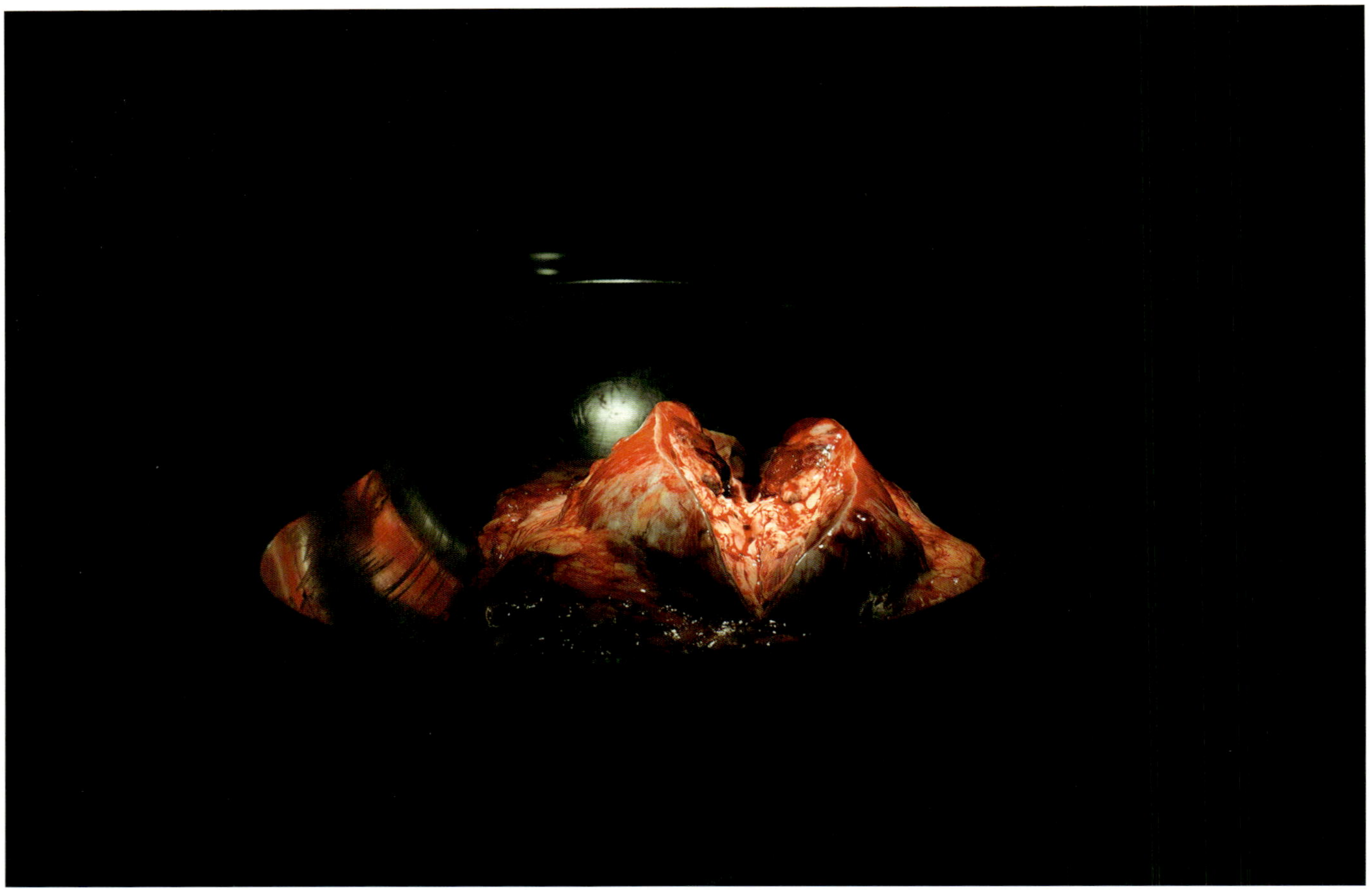

| SURGEON B | SURGEON A | SURGEON M |
|---|---|---|
| | *Ok, that one is split.* | *Something has been split right there.* |
| *That's cancer. Isn't it?* | | *Yep.* |
| | *Could this also be ovarian?* | *Could it be the uterus? That could be a myoma.* |
| *Yeah.* | | *Or what's over there?* |
| | *Very white for a uterus but I guess it could be it.* | |
| *It has a pretty strong capsule around it.* | *Indeed and then that could be like muscular that one.* | |
| *A kidney cancer. Yeah, of course.* | *A kidney. Okay. Well, they are both in the abdomen.* | |
| *But like M said, there's apparently a tumor there. This must have caused hematuria.* | *A split kidney.* | |
| *That's why the capsule is so strong. There's the cancer.* | *There's that fat, that's Gerota's fascia.* | *Yeah, okay.* |
| | *In hindsight it's easy to say that it's a kidney, but it does look somehow strangely white for a kidney.* | |
| *Does it look to you that this one was found in a relatively early state?* | *Still, quite a lump.* | *But then again, you can't see if it grows through the capsule...* |
| *So that the capsule would be intact.* | | *...and you can't tell if it grows all the way to the pelvis, or is it only there in the parenchyma.* |
| *Yeah.* | | |
| *There must have been hematuria.* | | *Yeah, or then again it could have been an incidental finding in some other screening.* |
| *So an unnecessary examination found this.* | | *Yeah.* |

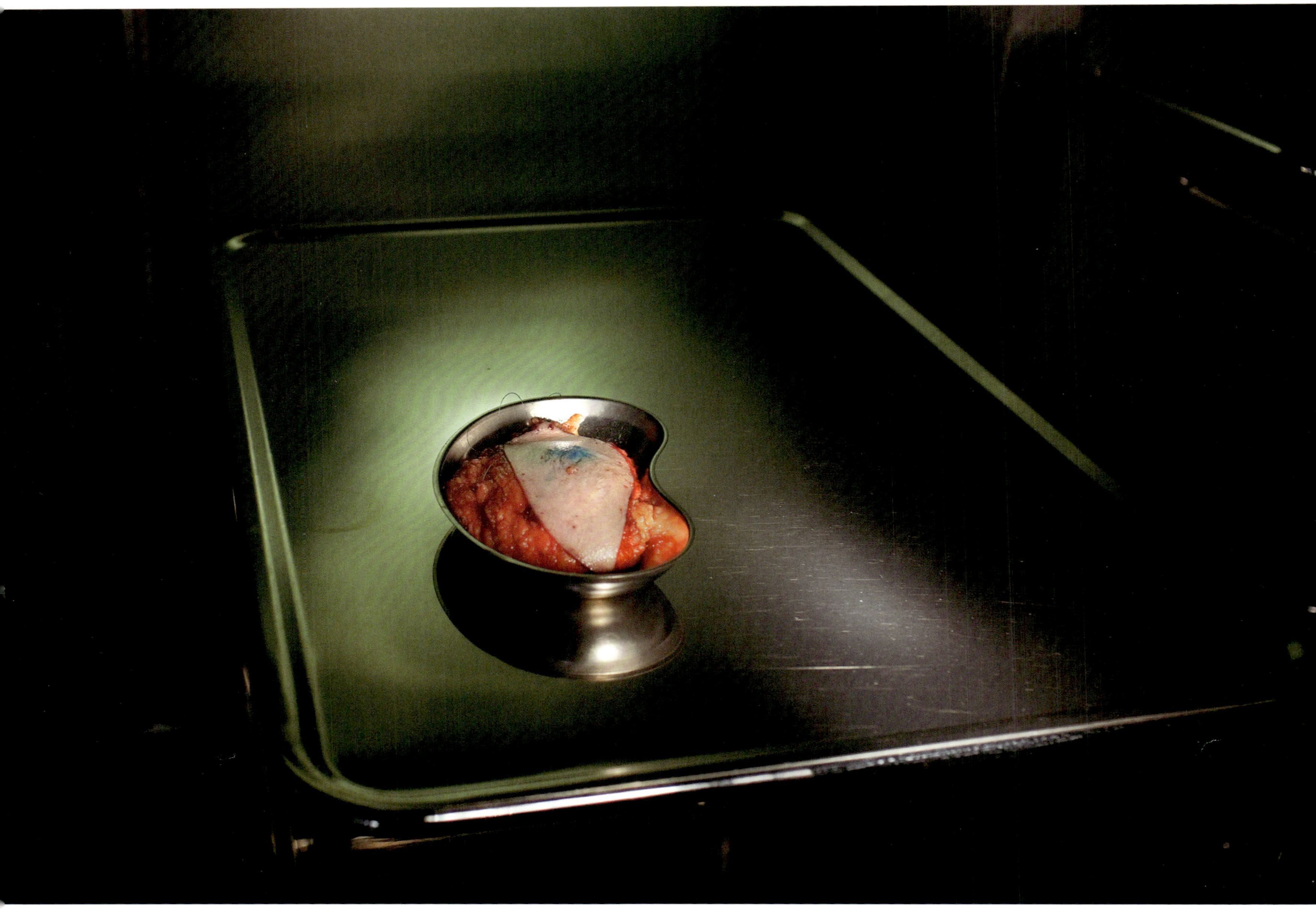

| SURGEON B | SURGEON A | SURGEON M |
| --- | --- | --- |
| | *Breast.* | |
| *Why is it dyed?* | *Well it's because they have dug up the sentinel lymph node. It's the same logic as with melanoma. You use that blue dye in the para-areolar parts there.* | |
| *Do you usually simultaneously use radio-activity also?* | *Yeah. That's just a tool.* | |
| | *Not everyone uses the blue dye but most still do, I guess.* | *Do you look for the primary tumor or just the sentinels with that?* |
| | *The sentinels.* | |
| *So here's...* | *So you don't put that where the tumor is but in the sector...* | |
| *Where the tumor is.* | *...here in the corner where the tumor is. So if it's an upper medial tumor for example, then the blue dye is put there para-areo-laric because that's where it spreads to the armpit the easiest.* | |
| *That's how you know where the drainage will be in the area.* | *Yes, yes, that must be the sentinel, but this is a total mastectomy too.* | |
| *So it would be a removal of the whole breast.* | *Yeah. A lot of fat and mammary gland tissue.* | |
| *You'll end up with very large raw surfaces when you remove this. Then interstitial fluids will seep through.* | *Usually they'll turn out just fine.* | |
| *At Hyvinkää we had a seroma clinic every Thursday. There were as many as seven people at its best. Or should I say at its worst.* | *And you went there and punctured seven boobs then?* | |
| *Yeah, well it was quite, you took it quite pragmatically. Just put the needle in and the serous fluids out.* | | |

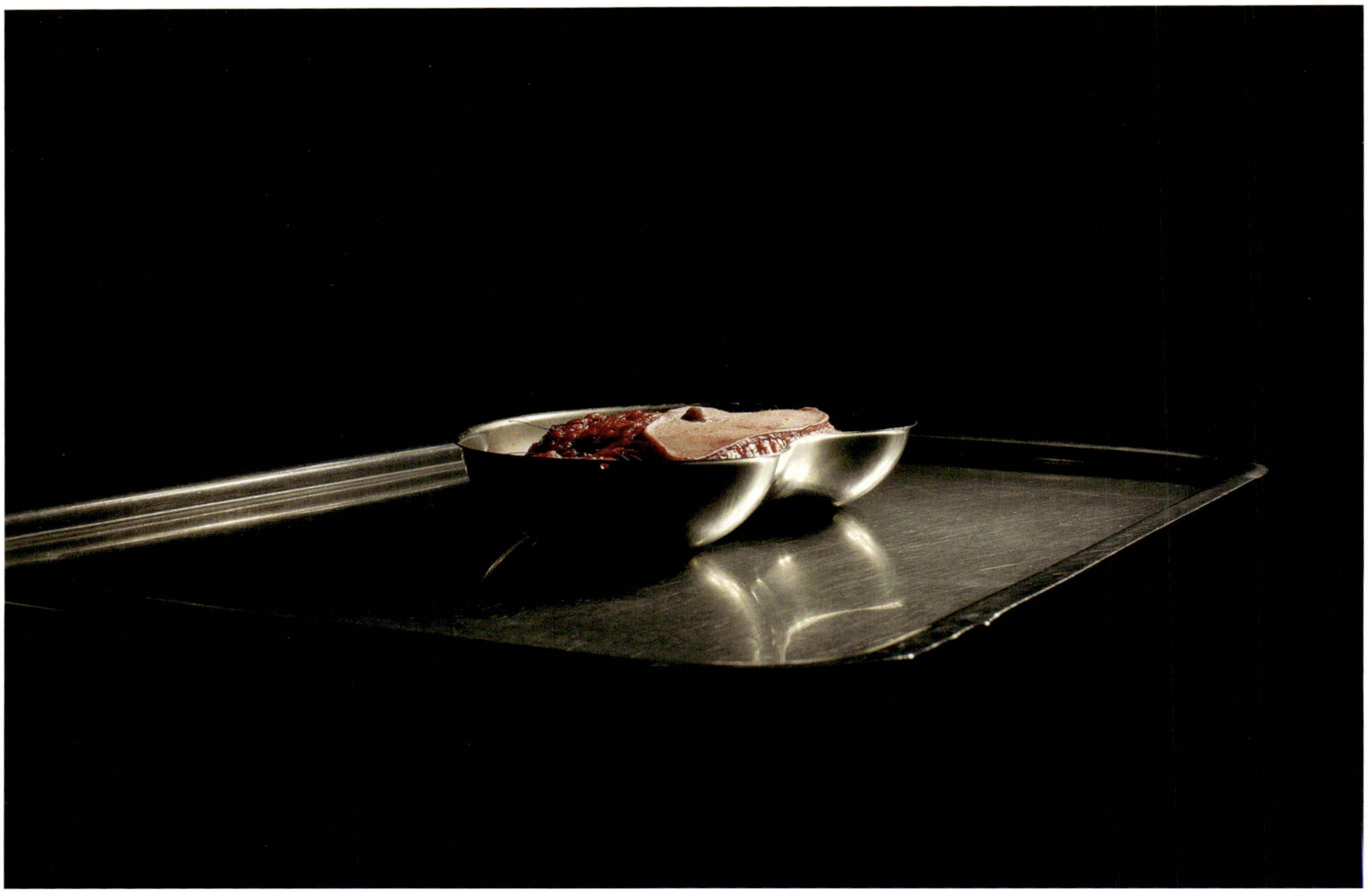

| SURGEON B | SURGEON A | SURGEON M |
|---|---|---|
| *Wow, this is a nice one. A hard looking boob.* | | *This is a big breast. It fills up the whole emesis basin.* |
| *This one has been eating a lot of butter and drinking whole milk.* | | *Yeah, not a small breast, but isn't this quadrantectomy or is that the whole...* |
| | *But there's the whole nipple at least. I'd say that this could be...* | |
| *Well, this isn't a quadrantectomy.* | *You wouldn't do a quadrantectomy if you remove the nipple.* | *Yes.* |
| | *It makes no sense.* | |
| *It looks like a metal butt and then there's the boob also.* | | *Well, there is a great amount of that, must be quite heavy...* |
| | *That breast must weight over a kilogram.* | *Yeah.* |
| *But this looks like the fat is very solid, doesn't it?* | | *Yeah, that's been a very firm breast indeed.* |
| *It's interesting how people's fats are so different. Some have very white and loose fat...* | *Quite dead looking fat and then some have quite, like, cadmium yellow, very...* | |
| *Dense, yeah.* | | *Some fat like, breaks into atoms when you grab it.* |
| | *It turns into powdered sugar.* | |
| *Once I got very, almost like, upset during an inguinal hernia repair when the patient had exceptionally white fat, very loose and wobbly. It was really uncomfortable.* | *But people with darker skin also have white fat.* | |
| *Really?* | *Yep.* | |
| *Why?* | *I think, it could be that somehow the cholesterol profile or something else is different? There must be a reason why it's different in color.* | |
| *You would imagine that it has an effect on one's health.* | *People with dark skin have white fat.* | |
| *Well, that's as white as it gets.* | | |

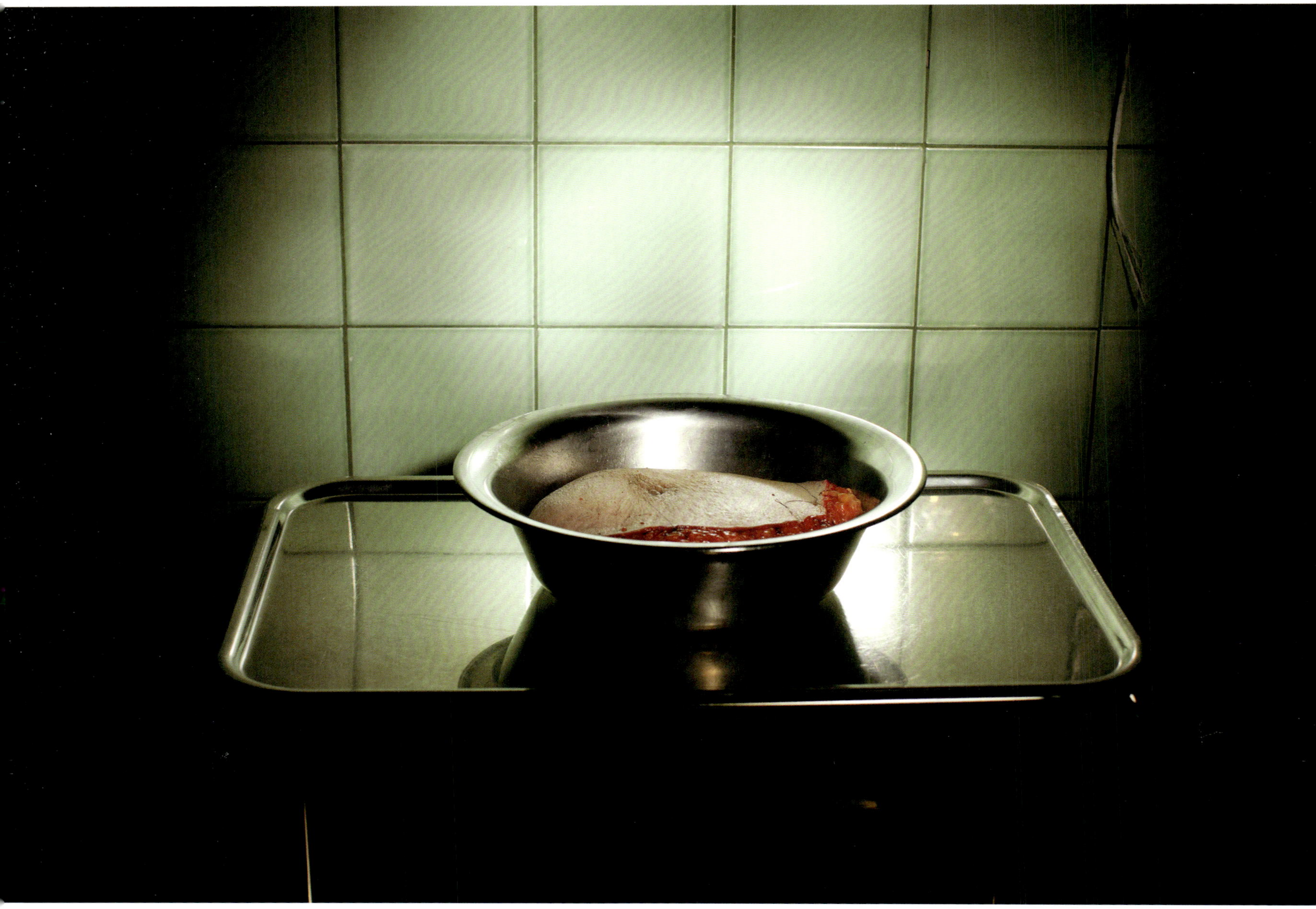

| SURGEON B | SURGEON A | SURGEON M |
| --- | --- | --- |
| | | *This is quite big.* |
| *Here you can see that the nipple has inverted. Could it have something to do with the tumor or could it be just because of the removal?* | *Maybe it is because of the removal. But it could also be inverted, of course.* | *This is clearly from someone older. They have removed a lot.* |
| | *Yes.* | *There's a lot of stuff.* |
| *It's very unpleasant to hold that kind of breast in your hand, in my opinion.* | *I think holding toes with arteriosclerosis obliterans would be even more unpleasant.* | |
| *Yeah.* | *That kind of black gangrenous toes.* | |
| *For me somehow, a breast is something vulnerable that you should like, protect and then you go and cut it out with a scalpel.* | *It's funny how you can think of it like that. I somehow take it extremely pragmatically. I don't have any emotional attachment to a breast.* | |
| | *(laughter)* | |
| *For me it's like, 'uh, disgusting'.* | | *I don't know, if it were my own breast there, I might have a different approach, but... breast is something that you can have removed without it making your life more difficult. You can rebuild it and...* |
| | *You can cut it out, like you can cut out your kidney or testis.* | |
| *They come in pairs.* | *Yes.* | *Indeed* |
| *You'll get along with just one.* | | *Or as for those you'd get a long without either one.* |
| | *Yes, you would, at least physically.* | |

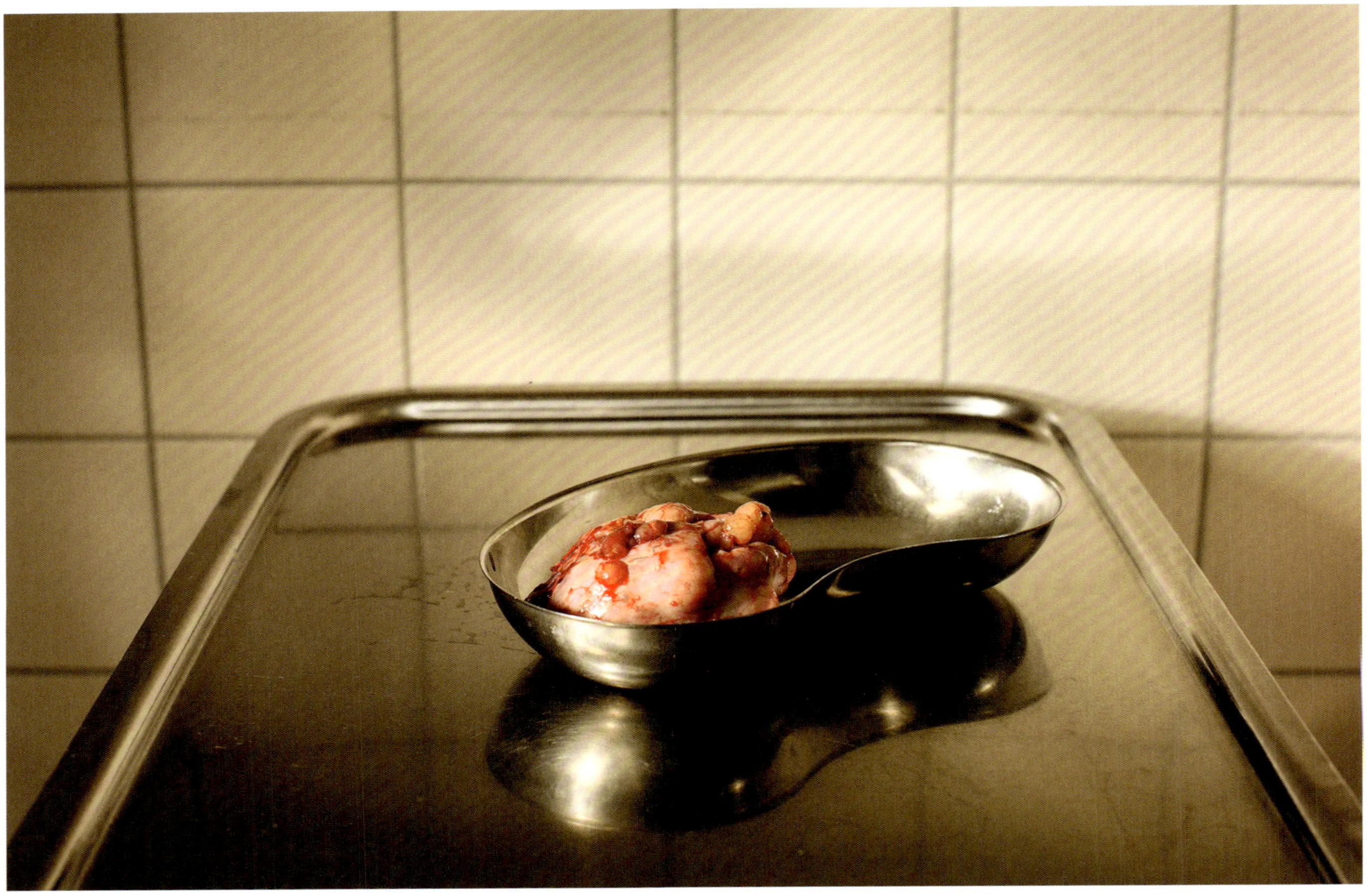

| SURGEON B | SURGEON A | SURGEON M |
| --- | --- | --- |
| | *Well, well.* | |
| *There's some...* | | *Well, this one is bigger than my fist. But what is it?* |
| | *It's a...* | |
| *Well, this is a big one.* | *Well, it isn't intestine anyway.* | |
| *No, there isn't anything like...* | *And this isn't the thyroid either.* | |
| *Quite big for a thyroid.* | *Well, it is very big...* | |
| *Could it, it isn't a kidney then?* | *Nope, not the spleen either?* | |
| *Not the spleen.* | *Nor... Umm. Oh, well. It's funny, I know it can't be it, but to me it looks like a cow heart.* | *I was just about to say that it looks a little bit like a heart but it's missing all the big arteries and...* |
| | *But it looks like a pump although it can't be one for sure.* | *What are these lumps here on the top?* |
| *Is this fat?* | | *Are these lymph nodes?* |
| | *It's too big for a thymus.* | |
| *Could it still be a thyroid, just a really big one.* | *Yeah, and why would anyone remove the thymus from a person?* | *If this could be a kind of thymoma or something?* |
| *Ovarian cancer.* | *Ovarian. Well, you can tell we're not gynecologists. We can't think of this stuff because we never remove them.* | *Yeah.* |
| *I guess these ones are pretty bad.* | | *Yeah, ovarian carcinoma. You can tell that it's something malignant, there are some strange metastases and...* |
| *This looks hard.* | *Firm.* | *That's cystic, at least partly a cystic ovarian tumor.* |
| *Yeah.* | | *Yeah, this might be the first one of these diseases that I wouldn't want for myself.* |
| *Yeah and all the rest you'd like?* | *You wouldn't want the ectopic testis either.* | *Yeah, well I wouldn't want that one either, but this is a nasty disease.* |
| | *(laughter)* | |
| | *Yeah, that's true.* | |

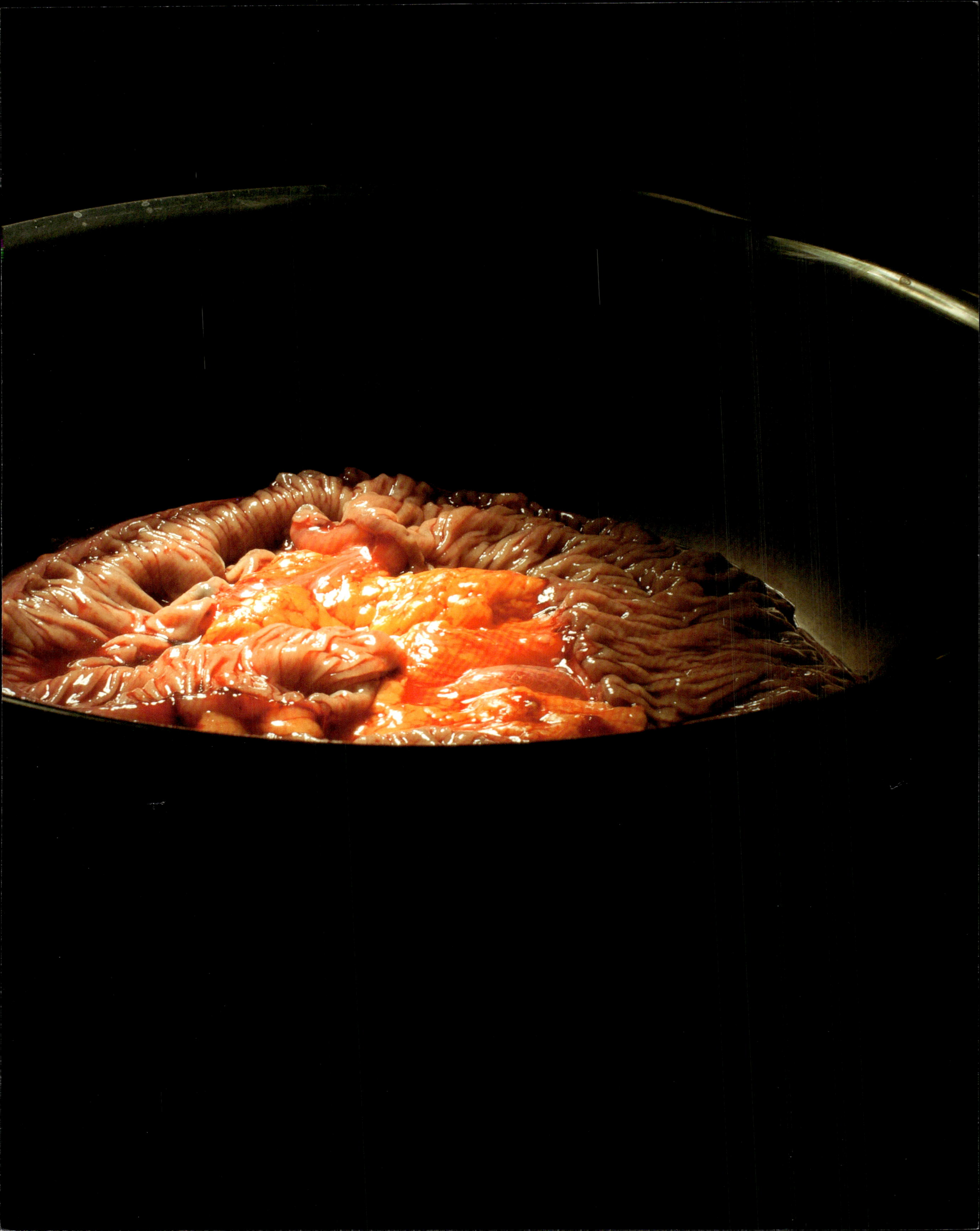

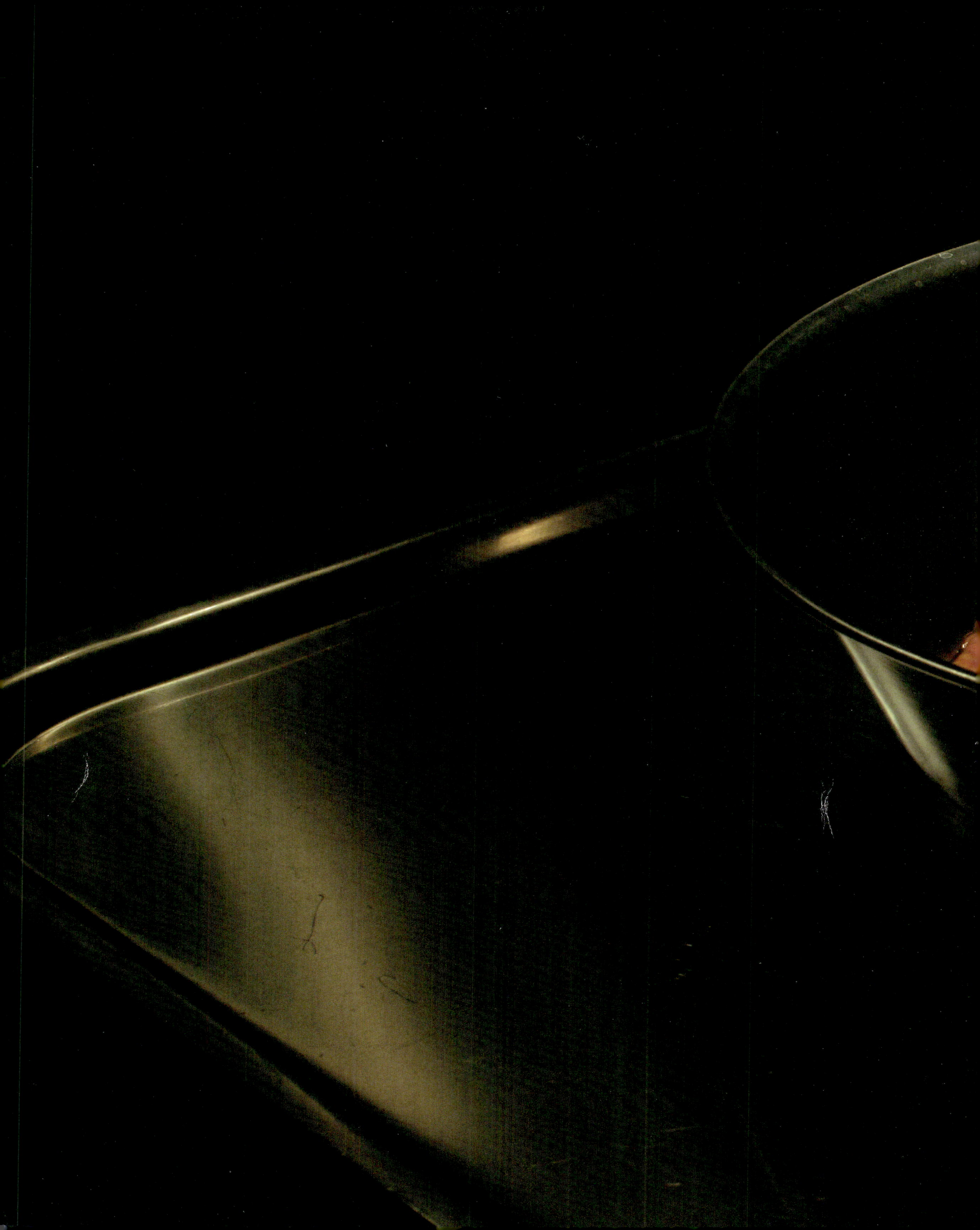

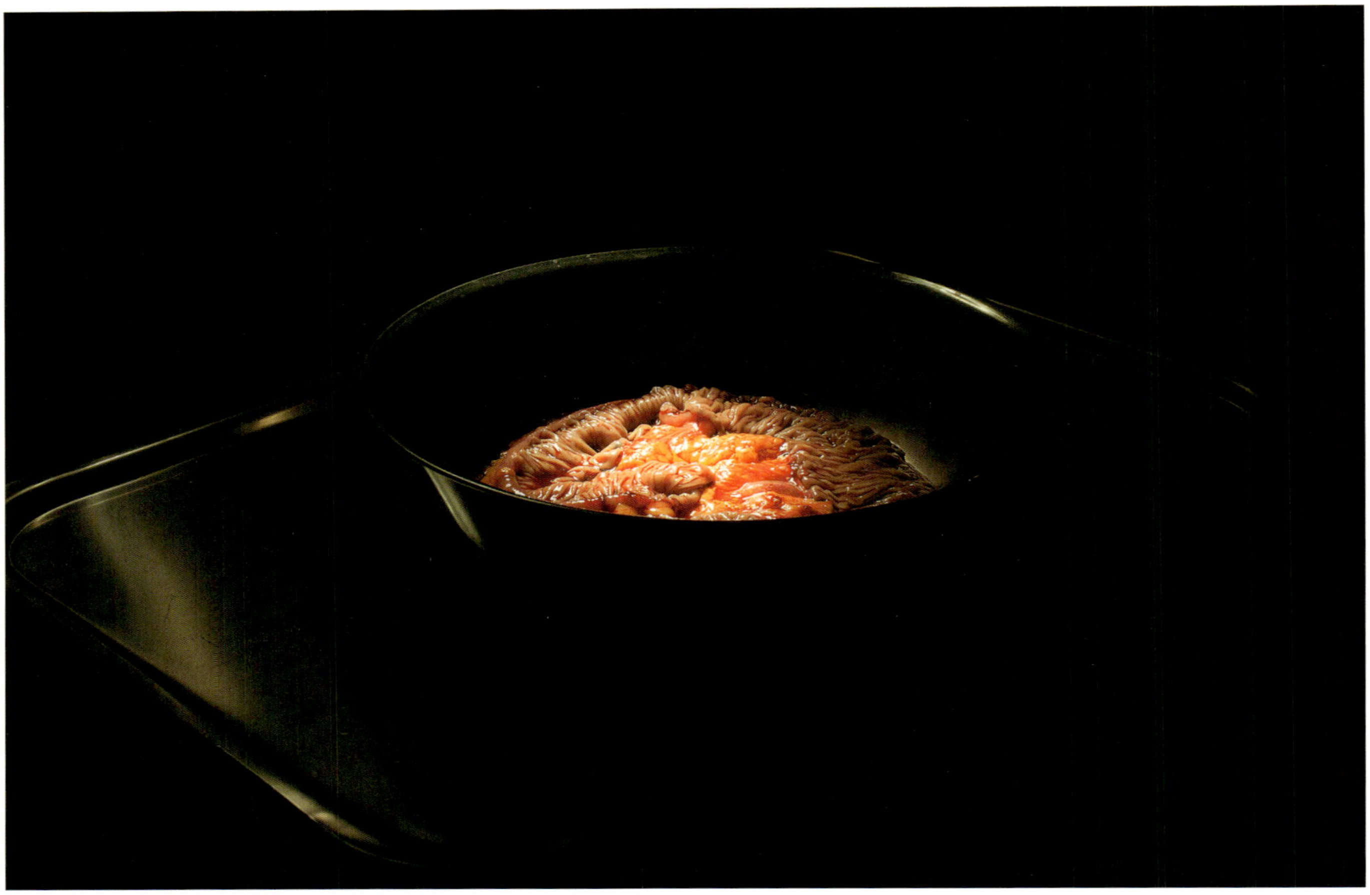

| SURGEON B | SURGEON A | SURGEON M |
|---|---|---|
| *This is beautiful. This is a nice one.* | | *Yeah, it's a part of the colon.*<br><br>*It's been opened there.* |
| *Is this colitis ulcerosa, because it's such a long bit?* | *You can't see the tumor there.* | |
| *This is a big basin, isn't it?* | *Yes.* | *So, is this colectomy then, or subtotal colectomy?* |
| | *It's funny how that mucous membrane goes around the outer rim there.* | *Can you see any tumor or ulcer or...* |
| | *Something.* | |
| *Could it be...* | *But it looks quite clean.* | |
| *It's clean all right, and there's nothing like an infection that you could see. It's pretty neat that in the colectomies, that are done because of colitis ulcerosa, there are these skipping lesions so that there can be a completely straight line after which the colon is affected. Have you seen those?* | | *I haven't.* |
| *It's strange how you can first have a healthy section suddenly followed by diseased one.* | | *Yes, Crohn's disease would look different.*<br><br>*I'm just trying to see if there's something in the meso or its fat, some lymph nodes or other things. There you have at least a few.*<br><br>*There could be...* |
| | *Some.* | |
| *What's the diagnosis here? Colon cancer, anyway. Where is the cancer?* | | *But somehow, they've removed a quite long bit then...* |
| *Because of the cancer.* | | *Yes.* |
| | *Is it some flat shaped adenoma, so that you can't quite...* | |
| *Maybe these are polyps all over here.* | | *Yes, if he's had some diverticulosis or something. Well, you can't see any diverticula either, but there must be some reason why there's so much...* |
| *Maybe he has a long intestine and constipation, so they removed a piece of transversum coli.* | *Yeah, you can a little...* | |

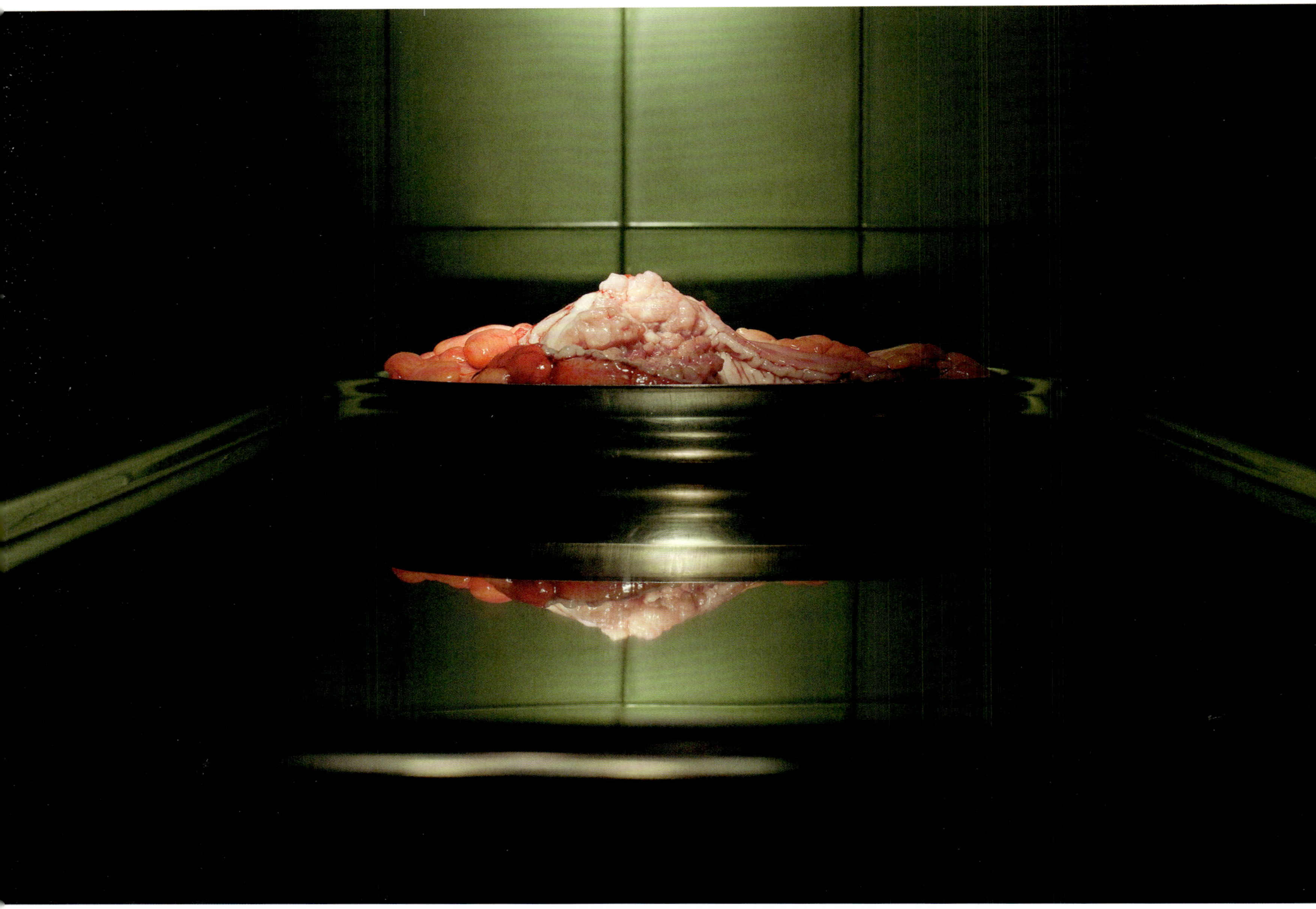

| SURGEON B | SURGEON A | SURGEON M |
| --- | --- | --- |
| | *This is intestine.* | |
| *And cancer, the real deal.* | | |
| *This is intestine cut open, must be the colon. Isn't that the colon, and a big tumor?* | | *So it seems.* |
| *There's the mucosa.* | | *Yeah, it's, see how it's wrinkled there, and...* |
| | *Serosa and mucosa.* | |
| | *That's a blocking tumor.* | *I would say that this is an intestine.* |
| | *It covers, like, the whole circumference.* | *This is some adenocarcinoma.* |
| *Looks quite nasty.* | *Is that the colon then?* | *I would say that it's the colon.* |
| | *I don't think anyone would...* | *No, that, that doesn't look like, the pattern of the small intestine, it doesn't fold like that, it looks different.* |
| *This layer just looks so thick, but maybe it is...* | | *That's a big tumor, like several centimeters.* |
| | *This is like, a bit like Mount Fuji.* | *Yeah.* |
| | *(laughter)* | |
| | *Yeah, isn't this just like a Japanese painting?* | |
| *A big plate of Frutti di Mare.* | | |
| | *(laughter)* | |
| | | *That's one of your own...* |
| | *Your very own colon.* | *...perversion.* |
| *I do tend to think about food quite often.* | *Colon frutti di...* | |

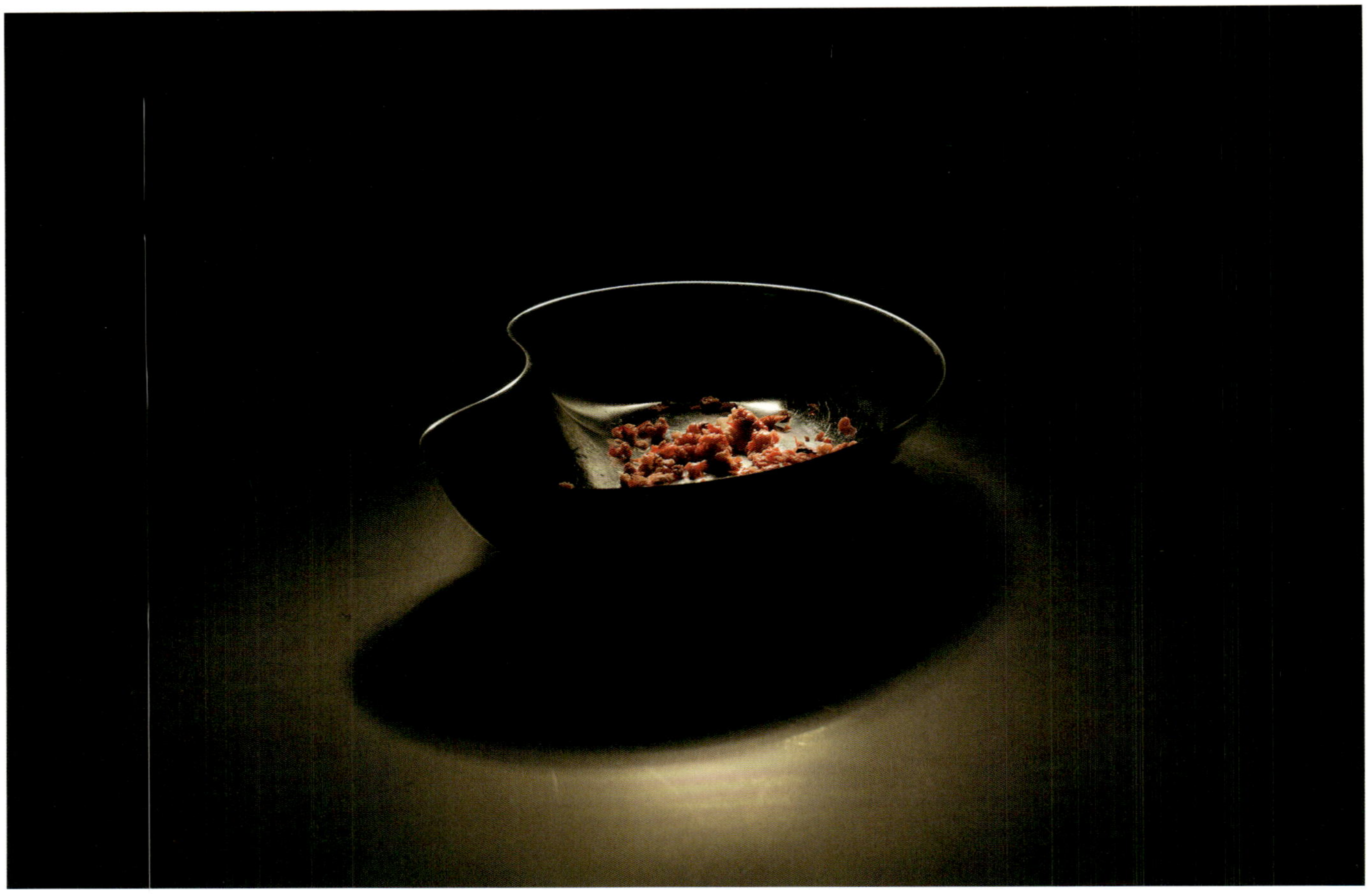

*And how much material there is from a hernia.*

*There's the one that's behind, that white could be it, but otherwise that's just discus and the bone that they gnawed out.*

*Yep.*

| SURGEON B | SURGEON A | SURGEON M |
| --- | --- | --- |
| *Some meatloaf.* | | *Okay...* |
| | *That's some fusilli and ground beef there.* | |
| *Looks rather delicious.* | *That's something, something plucked, or scraped or...* | |
| *A prostate.* | *No, these are too big...* | *These are flakes.* |
| | *Those would be a kind of whiteish brown, like beige colored. These are, there's blood on these.* | |
| *What are these?* | | *Are those snared from somewhere? Could these be some polyps?* |
| | *That would be hell of a lot, would anyone snare that amount of polyps?* | *You can snare them in three different sessions. This is a crazy amount though.* |
| *Could it be a resecate of the urinary bladder and then there's the big...* | *Could those be, umm, could it be vein... if they have plucked those...* | |
| *But there's no tubular structure.* | | *Yes, no tubular structure, and then you usually do get out some material that's possible to identify as a vein.* |
| *My guess is anyway that it could be something urological.* | *Now, are you telling me that it's not pasta bolognese?* | |
| *Spinal cord stenosis.* | | *Well, of course it is, there's some discus and bone.* |
| *Yeah, here's some discus.* | | *Yes.* |
| | *Yes, with Codman.* | |
| *Gnawed.* | *Yeah, they've been gnawed off...* | *Different sizes of bits with different equipment.* |
| | *Yes, Codman is the thing that, the big U-shaped jaws, that you can use to pick...* | |
| *(imitates the sound of the instrument) What's confusing here is that they have removed so much of it.* | | *Yeah.* |
| *He must have had bad symptoms or then they have removed it many times.* | | *But then again they might have done a laminectomy and gnawed out all other sorts of things so that isn't only waste from intervertebral discs there.* |

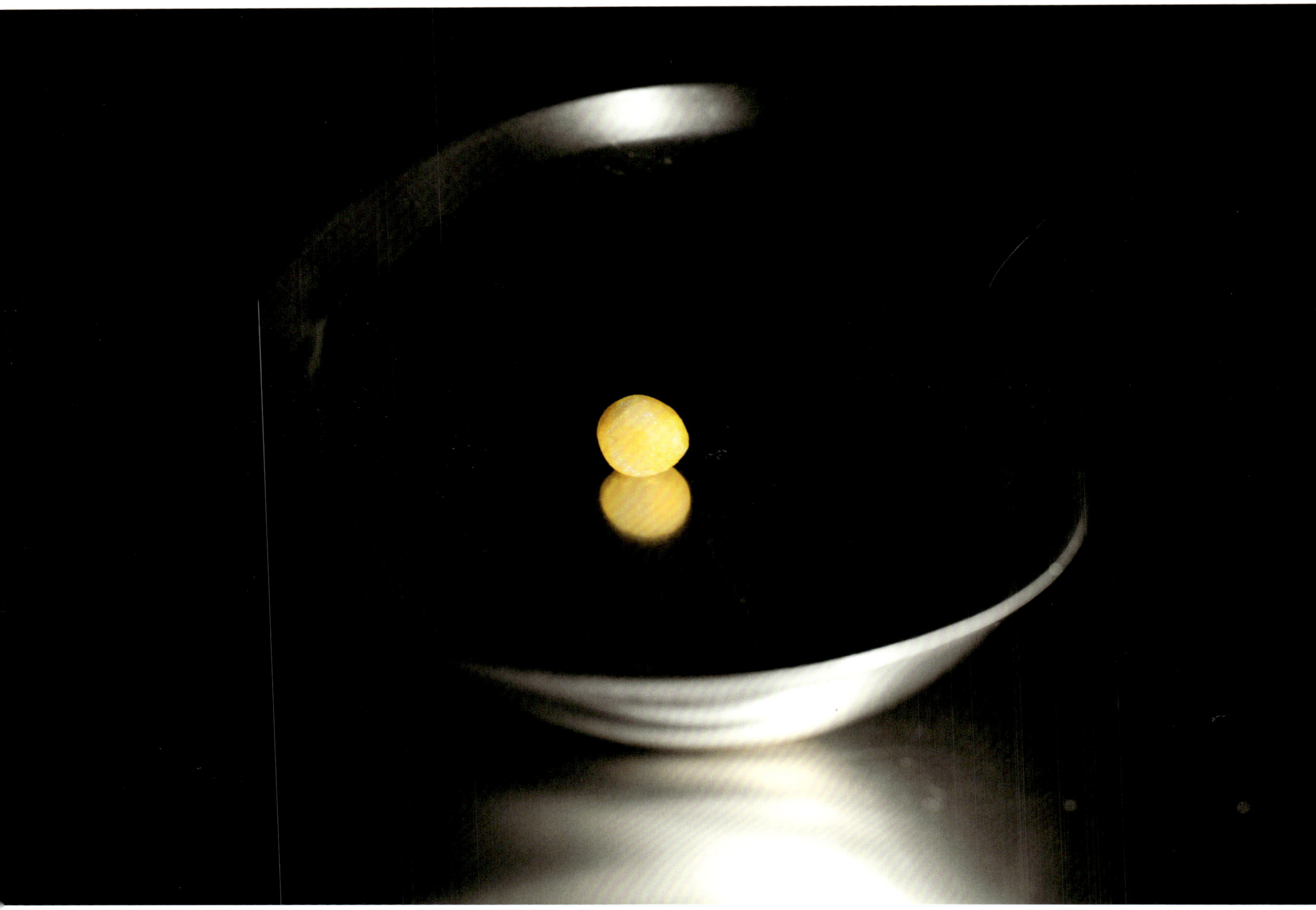

| SURGEON B | SURGEON A | SURGEON M |
| --- | --- | --- |
| *That's nice.* | | *Different etiology but it's a gallstone too.* |
| *I guess this is a cholesterol stone.* | *Yes it is.* | |
| *It can't be anything else.* | | *A nice yellow one.* |
| *It is a nice one.* | *It looks exactly like an astronomical object out in the Universe, because it's kind of like, a yellow globe.* | |
| *In a grey sterile environment...* | *Glowing like that. The emesis basin gives a halo effect.* | |
| *...glowing nicely.* | | |

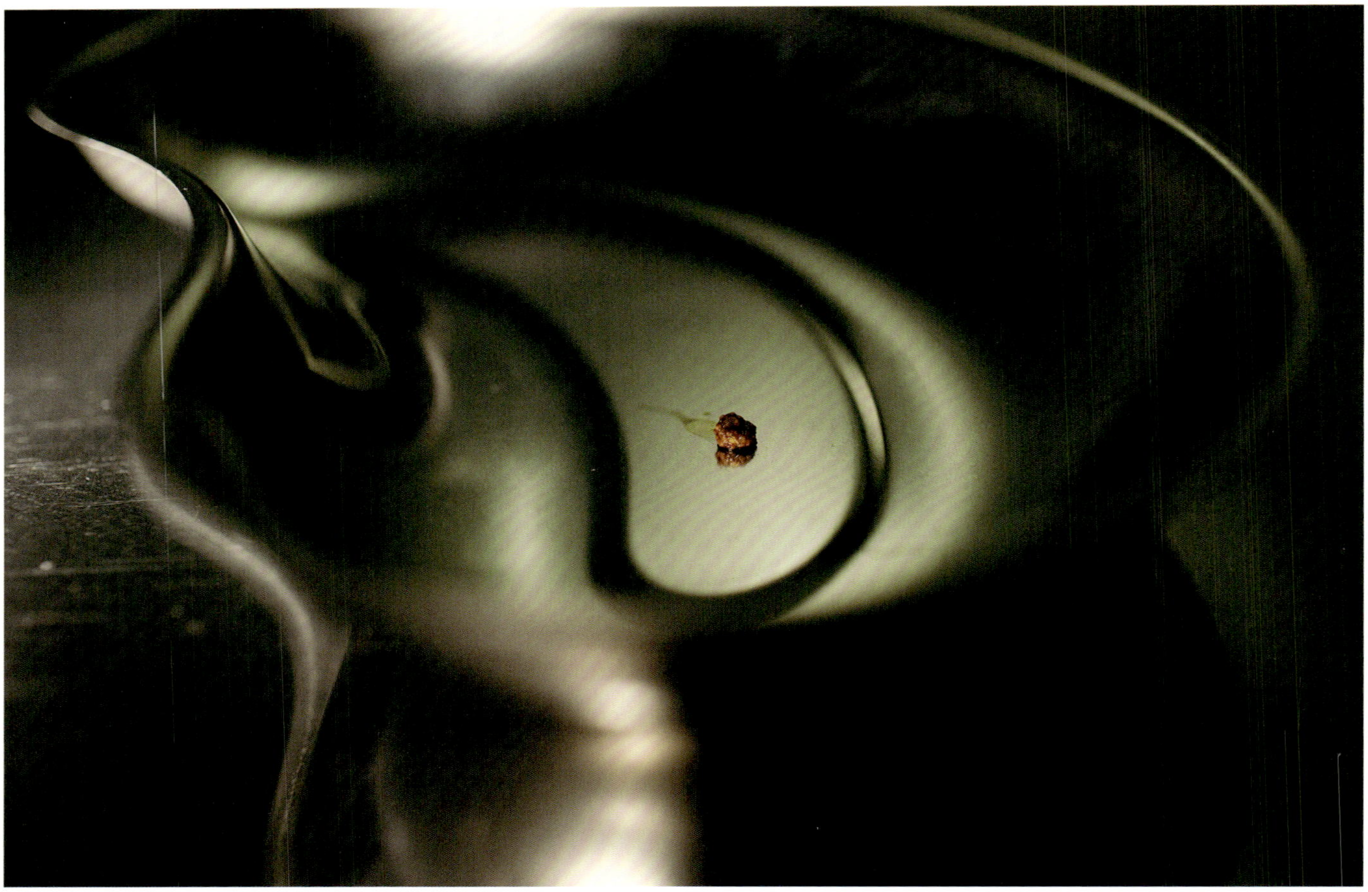

| SURGEON B | SURGEON A | SURGEON M |
| --- | --- | --- |
| | *A tiny one.* | |
| *'Plink.'* | | |
| *Is this a kidney stone or a cholesterol stone, a gallstone?* | | *Gallstone.* |
| | *Gall.* | |
| *It looks the same as...* | | *I'd say so, there's a trail of bile there behind.* |
| | *This is pathetic, compared to the first one.* | *Yes it is.*<br><br>*But it doesn't have to be big to cause a lot of trouble...* |
| | *Yes, a blocking stone.* | *It could be a blocking stone. Or cholecystitis, a removed one like this.* |
| *Yeah.* | | |

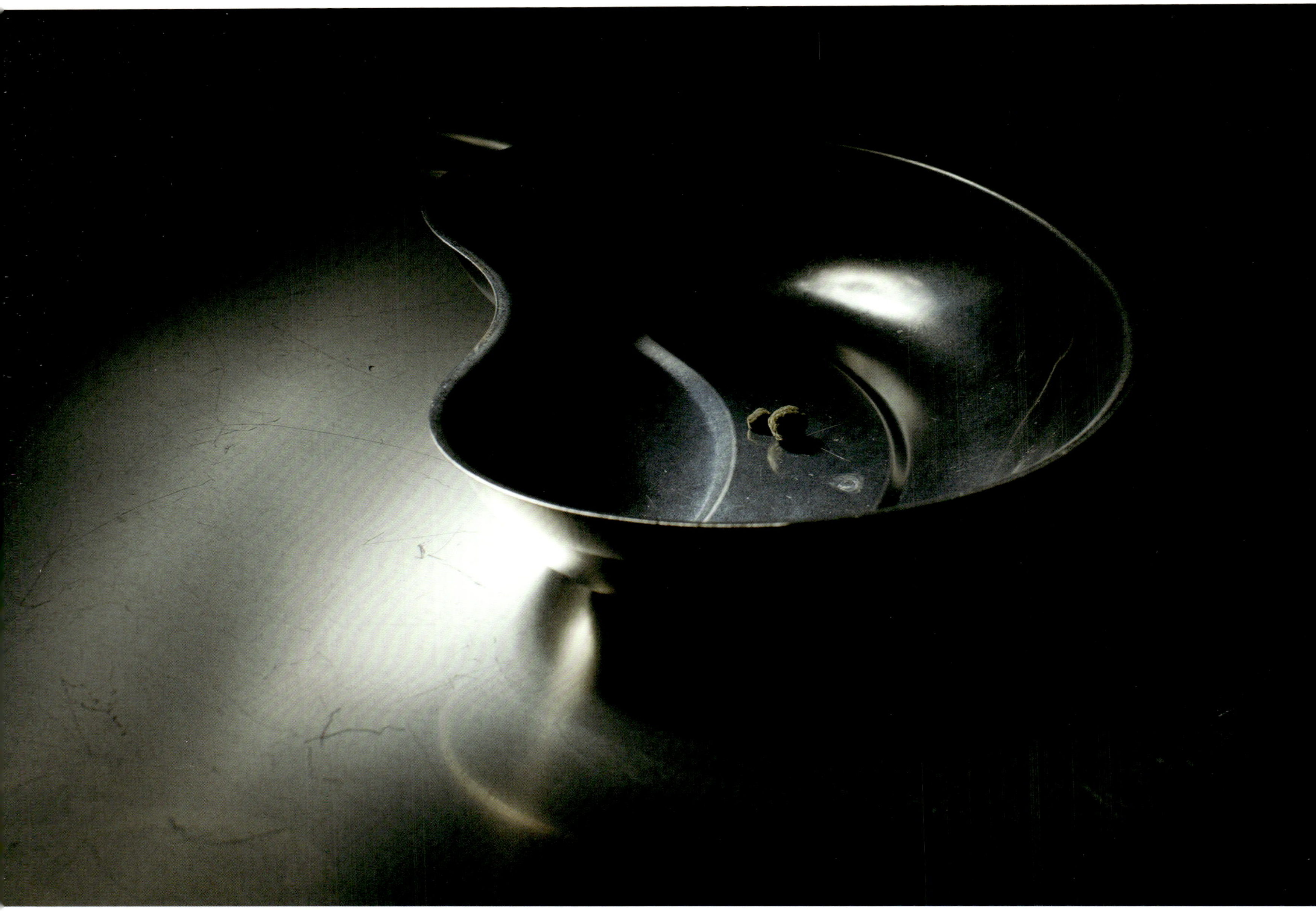

| SURGEON B | SURGEON A | SURGEON M |
| --- | --- | --- |
| *These look a bit pathetic.* | | *These are a bit ugly.* |
| | *Yes, these are a little bit gloomy. Look, the other one has, it has eyes, eyes and a mouth, it's like an alien.* | |
| *This is a bit like a moonlight view, like looking at the sky.* | *Yeah.* | *Yeah, these aren't nearly as sunny as the earlier one was.* |
| | *Well, these are some lunar orbs, if the earlier one was the sun.* | |
| *Yeah.* | *These are the brothers from the shadows. The shady brothers.* | *Not nearly as nice looking.* |
| *But these cause symptoms of course, these ones.* | | |

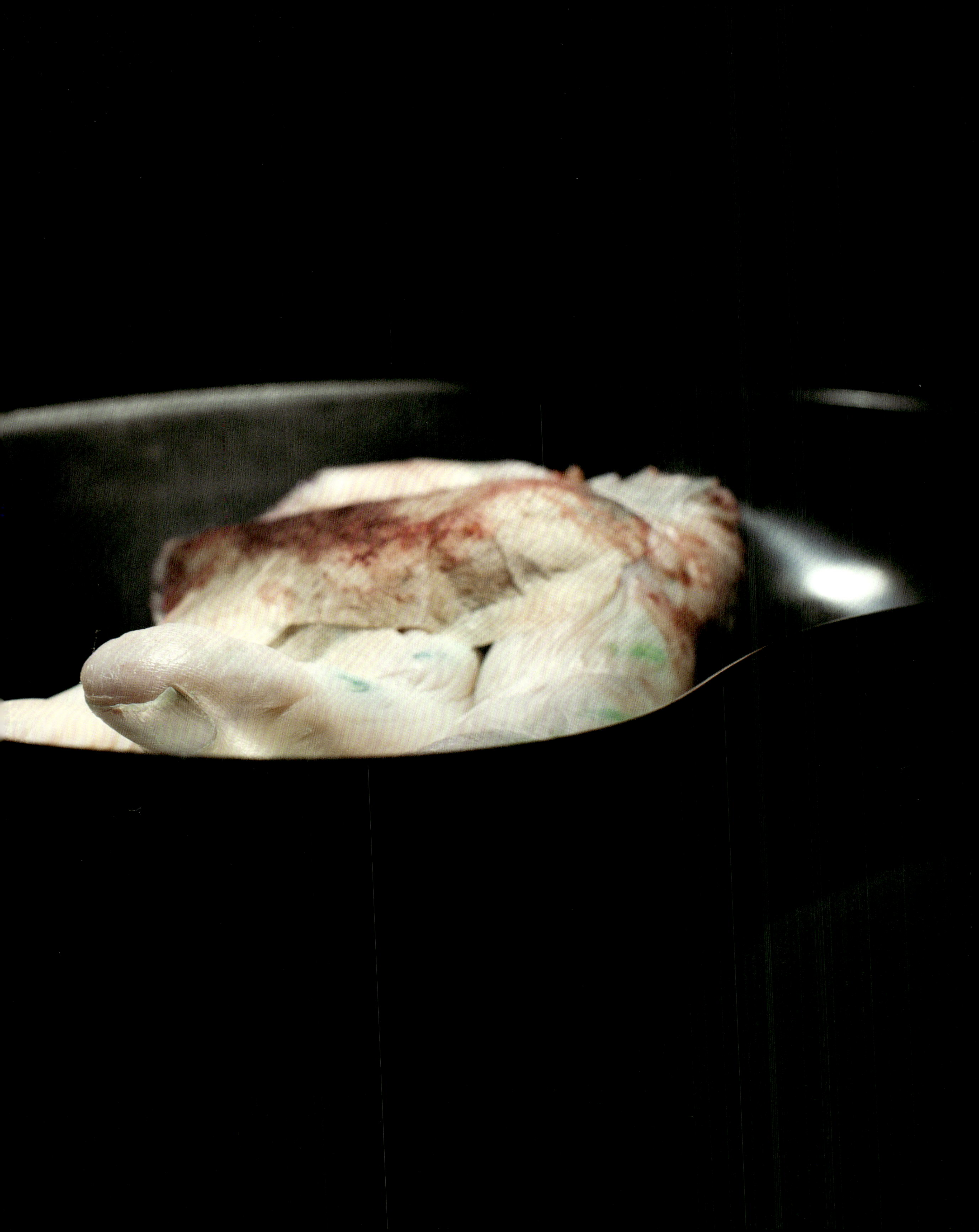

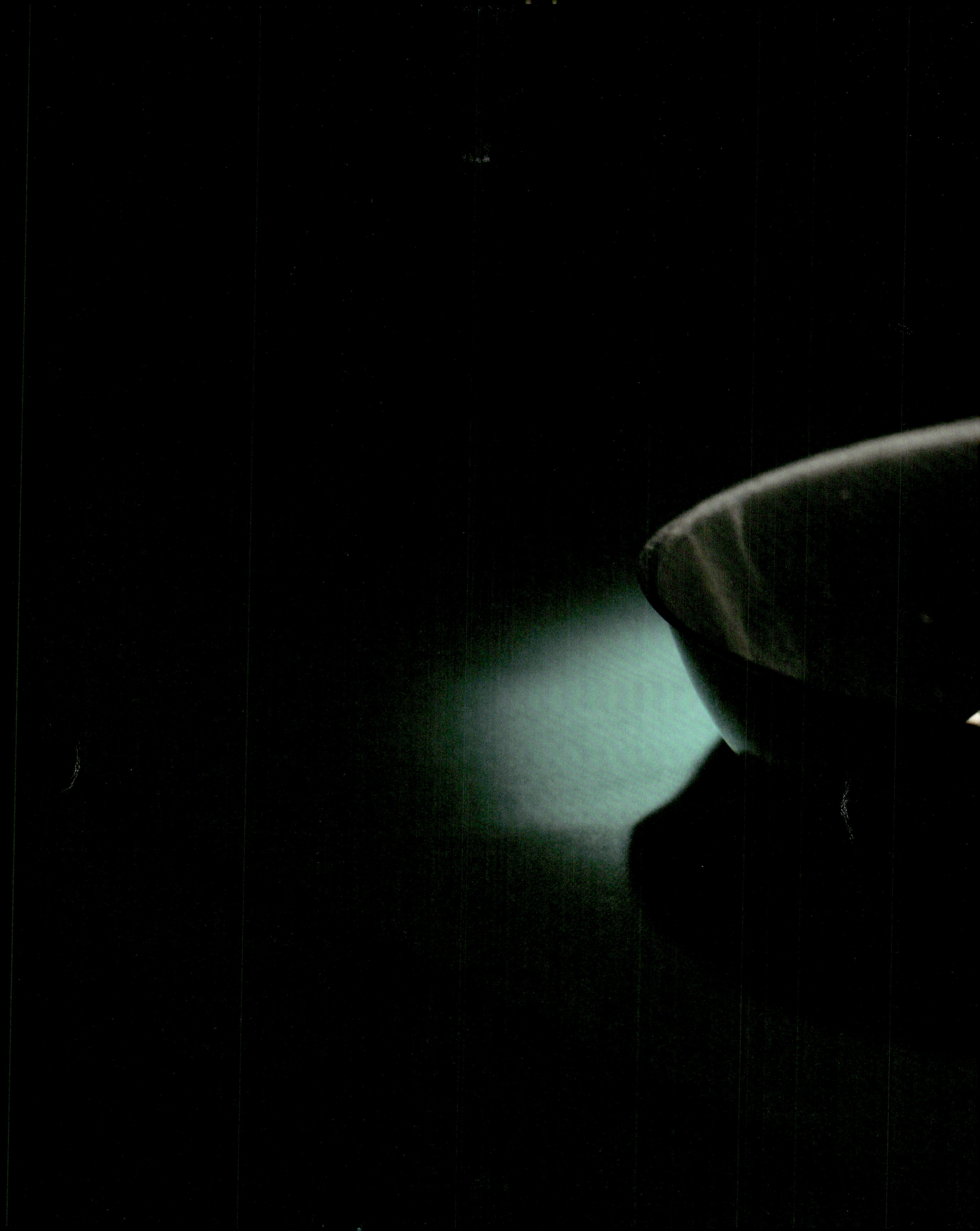

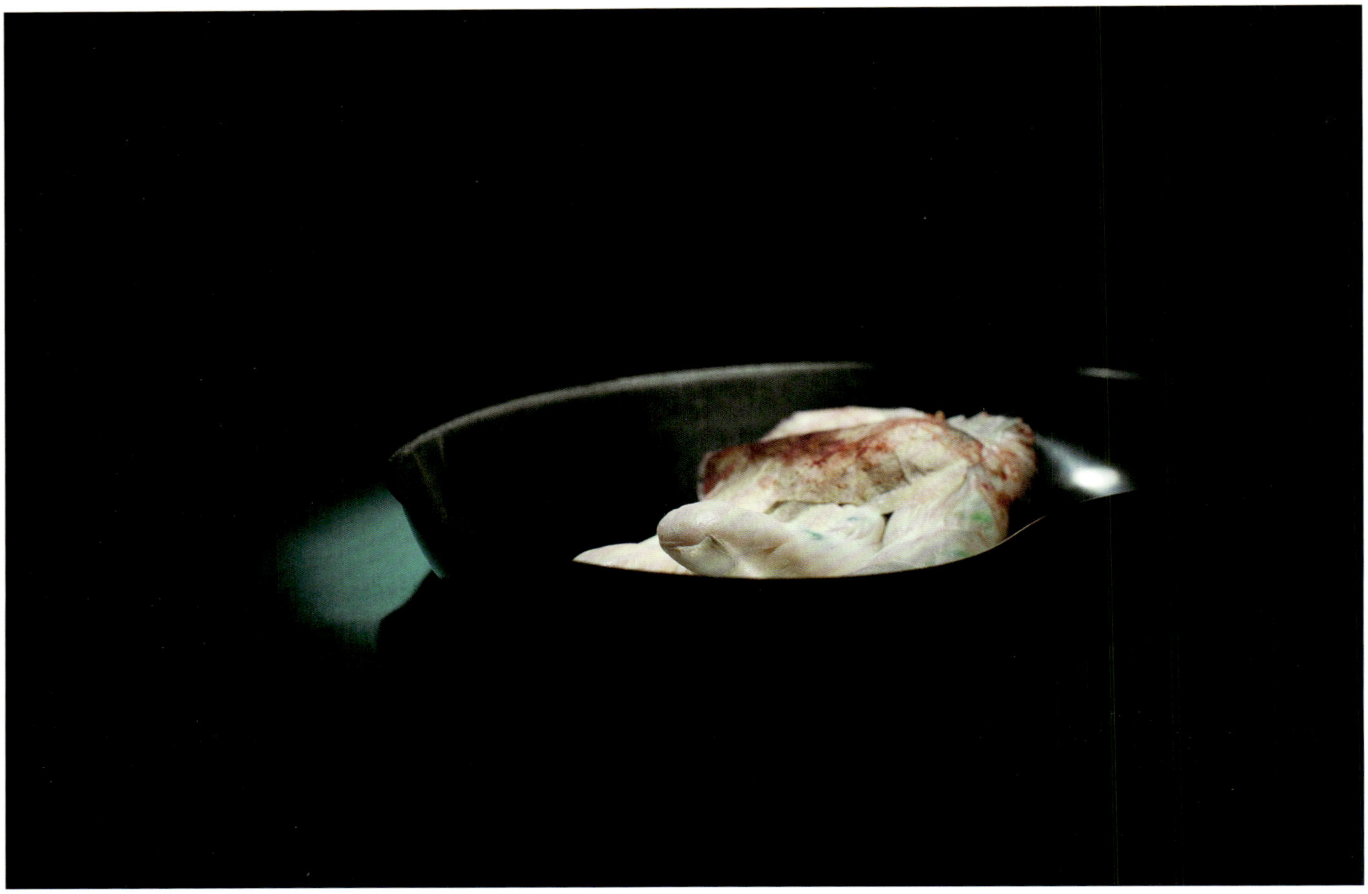

*You could imagine that the cancer has been here and that they wanted to preserve the little finger and the thumb.*

*Yeah, there you still have some kind of pinch grip left.*

*Yes, opposing fingers.*

*Now, which hand is this, is it the left one? Can you do it like this?*

*That's the three. But does that one look more like the second over there? It's hard to tell.*

*Yeah, you can't tell from that.*

*No you can't.*

| SURGEON B | SURGEON A | SURGEON M |
| --- | --- | --- |
| *Okay. Chicken fillet.* | *So it seems.* | |
| *Whoa, damn.* | | *Someone has lost a hand.* |
| | *Is it a hand or a toe? No, it must be a hand.* | *It's a hand.* |
| *A finger.* | | *There's like a...* |
| *A three.* | | *This is a three.* |
| *Now is this a traumatic amputation or is this because of cancer? There's some coloration here, what are those...* | *Could it be because of cancer after all, since there's that color and then some markings?* | |
| *But why would it be removed? There're at least one, two, three fingers at least.* | | *Three fingers. It looks like they would be these ones.* |
| *Would you remove so many fingers like this because of a cancer? Does it make any sense?* | | *I'm just trying to see if, the edge of the skin, it looks a little bad here...* |
| *Here it's ugly, the skin.* | | *...the skin. So could it still be some...* |
| *A trauma anyway.* | *Those fingers look clean, why would they...* | *Yes.* |
| | *...remove three fingers? It's crazy.* | |
| *Could it be accidental?* | *Yes, but what kind of accident?* | |
| *A circular saw.* | | *If something could have cut there for example, the skin is too neat for a circular saw.* |
| | *It looks dead, so white and glossy.* | *Well, there isn't much blood circulating in that hand at the moment.* |
| | *It's a bit like giving the finger there over the edge, so this one's just a little bit pissed off. It's like giving half a finger.* | *Cancer.* |
| *Okay, cancer. Why would you remove this?* | *Yeah, is it some bone cancer?* | |
| *Yeah, some sarcoma.* | *Or some connective tissue tumor, or, I don't know. This is a strange one.* | |
| *But this, this looks ugly. It looks like it's been peeling off.* | *There're markings so maybe they have planned it somehow, so that this would be removed, they haven't just sliced up the hand for fun.* | *Yeah, and that cut there is too clean to be a traumatic.* |

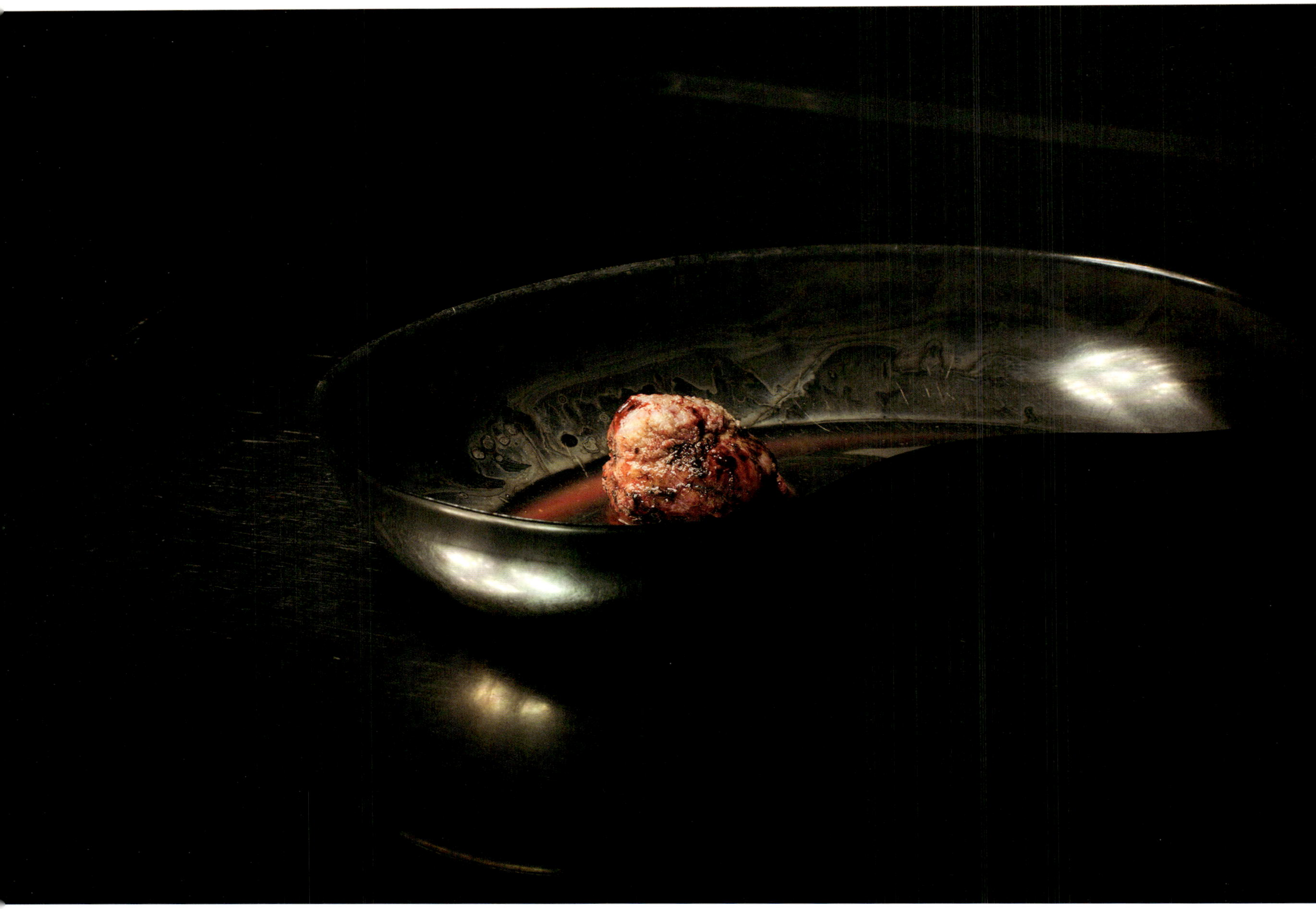

*Or almost the size of your prostate. Where your third brain resides.*

*Thanks a lot.*

*Scraping the brain.*

*(laughter)*

| SURGEON B | SURGEON A | SURGEON M |
|---|---|---|
| *Okay, what is this? Is it a tongue or what the heck is it?* | *Very rough surface.* | |
| *Is there some cancer there? Is it...* | *It must be a tumor.* | |
| *Is it a tongue?* | | *A thyroid? Could it be?* |
| *I mean, look at that surface, I don't know...* | *Usually you can recognize the capsule. Is that a thyroid?* | |
| *Brain tumor. Wow, we haven't seen that yet, have we?* | *No, at least I have never seen one.* | *Me neither.* |
| *It looks almost as if...* | | *Is there some brain tissue? Or have they just cut close by the surface of the tumor...* |
| *Or is it like, could it be meningioma?* | | *No, it would be surrounded by a kind of capsule. Isn't the only problem with meningioma that it causes pressure?* |
| *Yeah.* | | *But this one isn't, the surface isn't nice and neat. That looks more like it's growing from there.* |
| *Then it means that they took it with almost non-existing margins.* | *But then again, don't those neurosurgeons cut it like, quite, you know. I have understood that hemostasis is operated on aggressively, so that the surface is left pretty burnt up.* | *Well, they have done hemostasis here, because the surface is very black, here and there.* |
| | *I didn't even think of it being something from inside the head.* | *Neurosurgery is like a foreign country to me.* |
| *That is quite big one. You could imagine that it causes symptoms.* | | *Hmm.* |
| | *That lump is a sizable percentage of the brain.* | |
| *At least of my...* | | *Yeah.* |
| *...brain.* | | |
| | *(laughter)* | |
| *It must be a hundred grams.* | *Almost the size of your other brain, the testicle.* | |
| | *(laughter)* | |

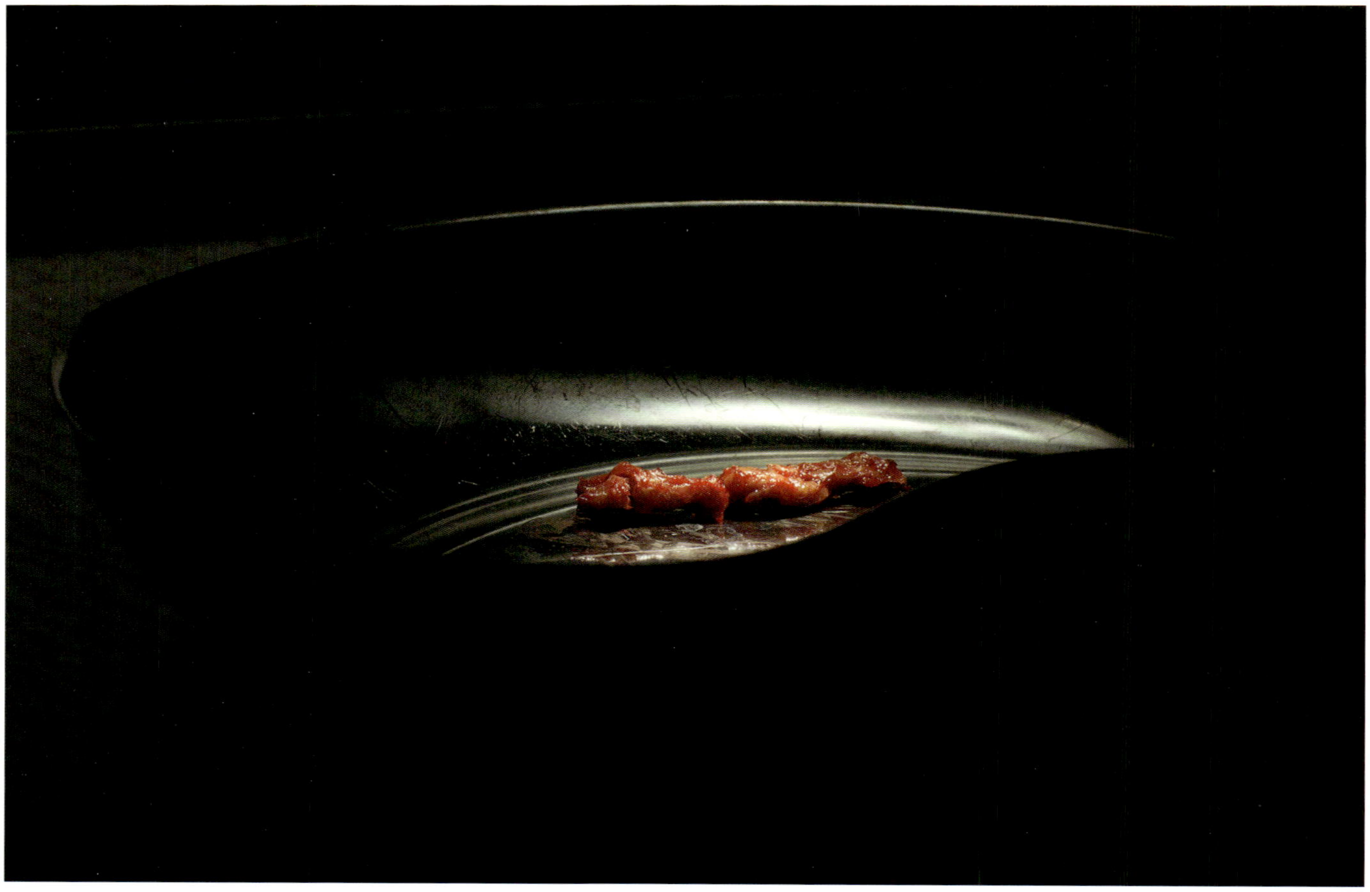

| SURGEON B | SURGEON A | SURGEON M |
| --- | --- | --- |
| | *No idea what it is.* | *Hmm...* |
| | *Oh.* | |
| | *(silence)* | |
| | | *That's like a grilled sausage, I just ate one.* |
| | *It looks very much like one. I really don't know.* | *It's quite, long-ish...* |
| | *Is there... there's not a vein here, is there?* | *No.* |
| | *And it isn't a thyroid either.* | *And those aren't testicles.* |
| | *Nor the ovary, uterus, or intestine.* | |
| *Is it a fistula?* | *It looks just like fat and...* | |
| *What size is this? It's in the emesis basin, just...* | | *On the bottom of the basin, just a few centimeters...* |
| | *Could it be lymph nodes?* | *Could it be a lymph node biopsy?* |
| *Atherosclerosis. Oh!* | | *They've done endarterectomy.* |
| *There you can see how stiff the artery is.* | *Yes, quite right.* | |
| *Really stiff.* | *That was a difficult one.* | |
| *A very interesting one.* | *Yeah, not suitable for a first timer.* | |
| *Nice one.* | | *If you can say something about that, it would be that it's not healthy tissue.* |
| *Yeah, it looks like barbecued meat skewer.* | *Yeah, skewered meat.* | |

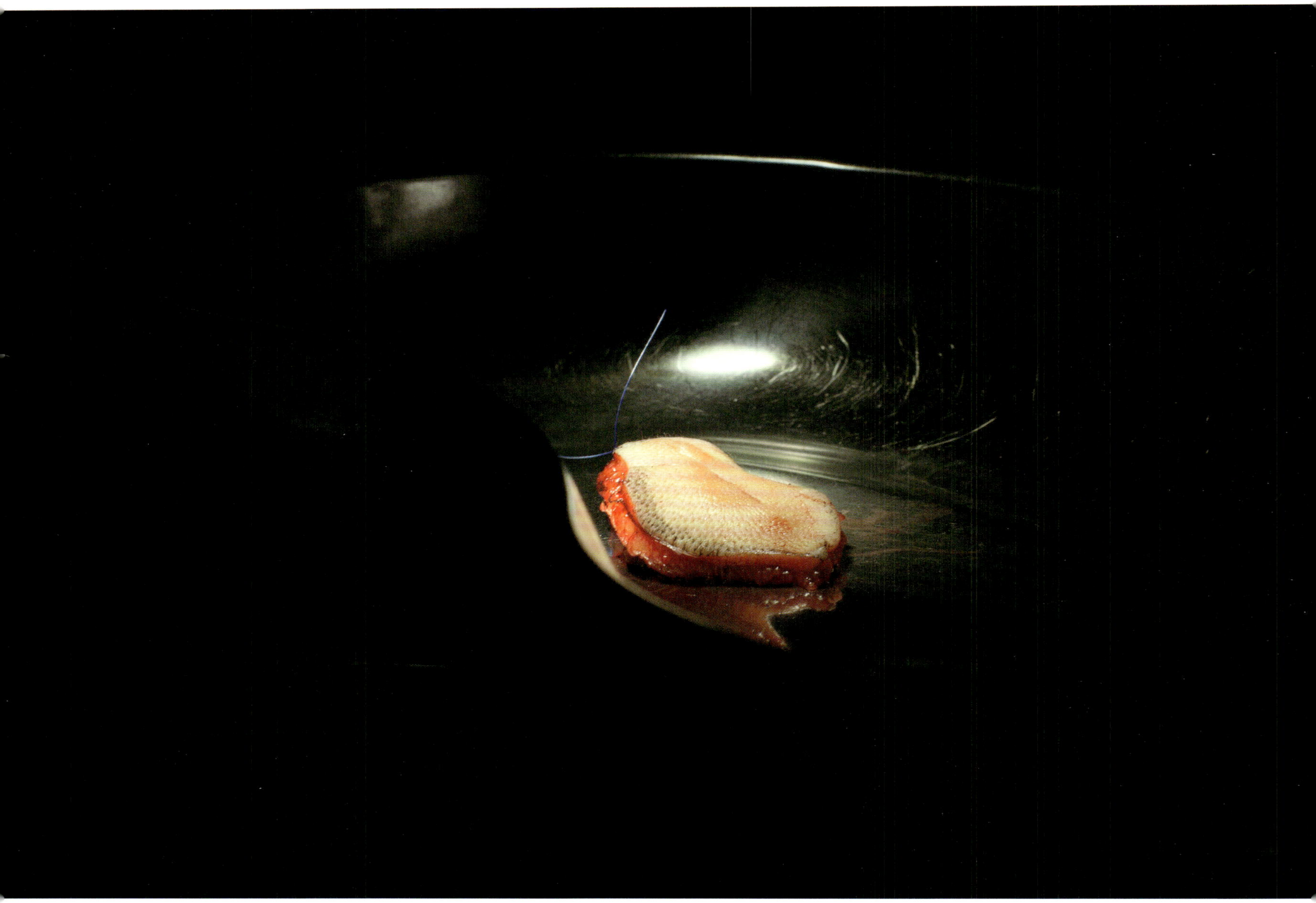

| SURGEON B | SURGEON A | SURGEON M |
|---|---|---|
| *This looks beautiful, this surface.* | *This is like pork skin.* | |
| *Or if you look at it like from a distance, it looks almost like salmon or...* | *Yeah, there's a scar in the middle, isn't there?* | |
| *Yes.* | *First I thought there was a sinus pilonidalis, I though there was a butt crack, but it's not a butt crack.* | *Could it be an additional resection of melanoma or some other...* |
| | *There's a suture.* | |
| | *And they have even done markings.* | *It must be something malignant. Is it, there's the fascia of Scarpa. Is this all the way to the fascia then?* |
| | *Or then it's somewhere in a thinner area.* | *What's that darker mark there, is it just some...* |
| | *Is it just some blood? Or is there something else on the edge, a skin mole? No, it's not a mole...* | |
| | *Yes, but this is some additional resection.* | *Soft tissue tumor of the back.* |
| *Ok, they took it with quite big margins.* | | *They might have taken some biopsy. Is the scar from a biopsy or is it something else?* |
| *A long biopsy scar.* | *Yes quite long indeed.* | |

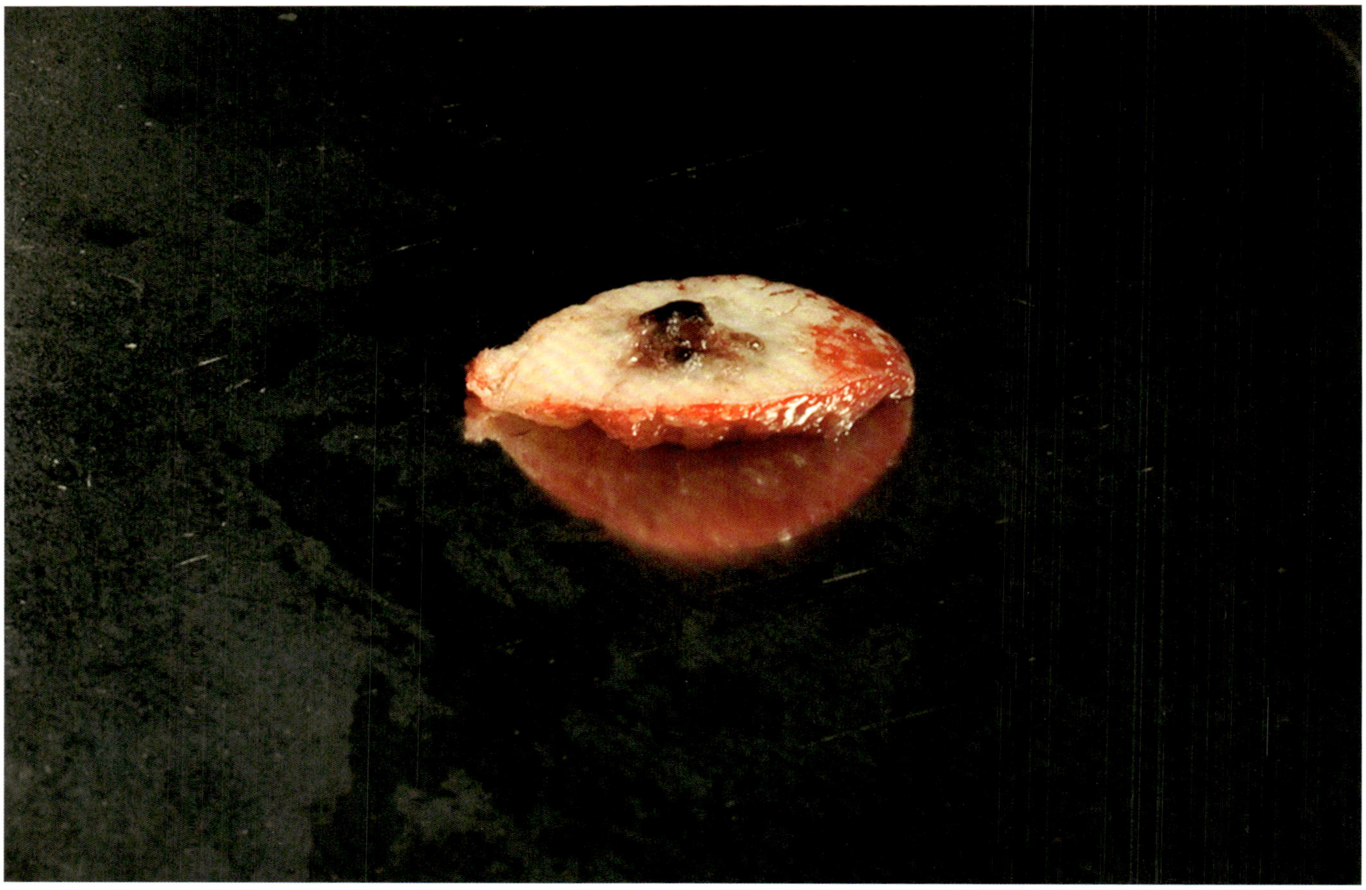

| SURGEON B | SURGEON A | SURGEON M |
| --- | --- | --- |
| | *Now, that is some kind of skin tumor.* | *Melanoma.* |
| *Yeah, nasty.* | *Or could it be just some scabbed...* | *They left quite small margins.* |
| *Yeah.* | *Yes, scabbed spinalioma?* | |
| *It's growing almost to the border.* | *That must be just basal cell carcinoma, if there's a scab. Or some benign tumor. Because melanoma would have more margins, they would have taken it all the way to the fascia.* | *That's taken only down to the fascia of Scarpa, that one.* |
| | *The dermis is quite thin so it must be an old person's skin.* | |
| *Yeah.* | | *It's not on a limb unless it's a thigh...* |
| | *Could it be head, face or...* | *Other parts don't have so much subcutaneous tissue. Quite heavy on that...* |
| *Cheek.* | | *I don't think that skin is, it's a bit like...* |
| | *I don't know.* | *It's hard to estimate the size here.* |
| *The skin looks quite greasy somehow.* | *But it can't be a melanoma. I think it's something smaller and less dangerous but there's just more scab.* | |

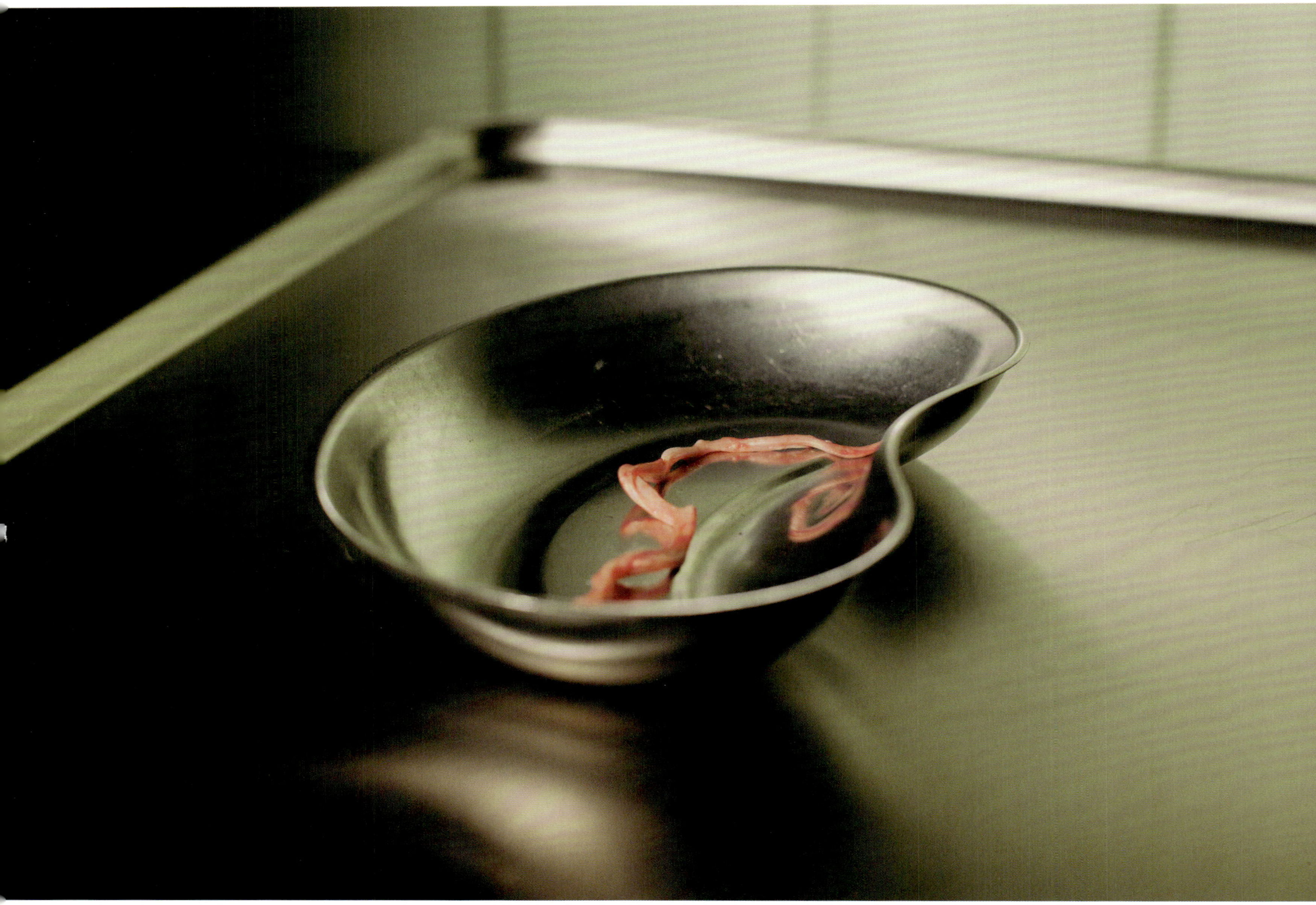

| SURGEON B | SURGEON A | SURGEON M |
|---|---|---|
| *What is this then? No...* | *A worm. It looks just like an earthworm.* | |
| *It looks kind of like a fish.* | *An earthworm! Just look at that. There's its saddle.* | |
| *What this is, is...* | *Now this is a blood vein.* | *But is it a vein?* |
| *Is it an endoprosthesis? What's over there? There's a sort of...* | *I don't thinks so, not in such a small vein. That one in the emesis basin, that's not a big one, it's just a few millimeters...* | |
| *Why is there like a regular...* | | *Fishnet pattern.* |
| | *It's a snake vein.* | |
| *Yeah, it looks like a skinned snake.* | *It does. The answer is a skinned snake.* | *I'd say that this is a vein.* |
| *A varicose vein.* | *So a varicose vein then.* | |
| *Where does this pattern come from?* | | *Could it be that it was grabbed it with some...* |
| | *With pincers.* | |
| *Yeah.* | *Yeah, with crile forceps!* | |
| *Yes!* | *With crile, yes of course. The gripping surface on crile, it has a...* | *Something must have made that pattern.* |
| *They've grabbed it and inched it out...* | *Yes, you've caught it from the other end and pulled like this. Then you started to wiggle it out. Quite a catch.* | *A good catch.* |
| | *I don't get big ones like this.* | *But has this one been removed with an open technique so that those branches are ligated? Is it removed openly, because would anyone... Or if it would be stripped, would it look like this either?* |
| | *And that would be upside down then, or like, inside out.* | *Yeah, isn't this exactly the right way then.* |
| *Is there some instrument inside it or why is it so stiff? Maybe it just looks like it. Look how it's rising up there. A vein is usually like jelly.* | *A varicose vein, deformed valves and...* | |
| *They are scarred.* | | *But aren't those loose too. I don't know.* |
| | *Funny, it looks very static. I wonder if it's dried up or something.* | |

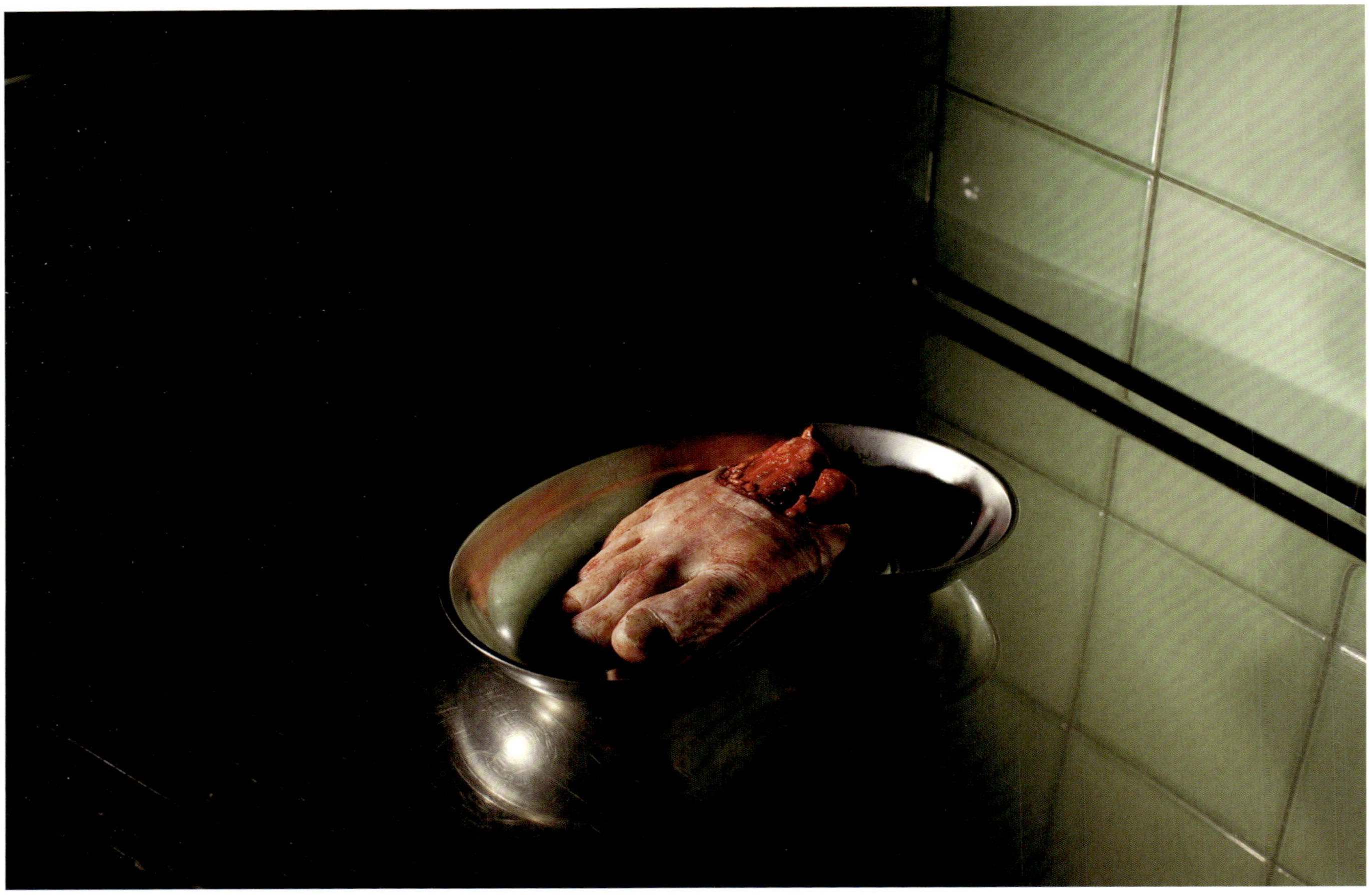

| | | |
|---|---|---|
| *I could imagine that this foot is completely numb.* | *Will he be happier with the metatarsal stump then?* | *Well, if it's a good stump?* |
| | *Right.* | *Yeah, this doesn't look that deformed.* |
| | *Yeah, it looks surprisingly neat like this. Usually they are like, if it's black, there're a couple of mummified toes, then it's obvious.* | *Yeah, then it'd be arteriosclerosis obliterans.* |
| *Maybe they took off the wrong foot?* | *Yeah, it was the other foot that was diabetic, not this one. Diabetes of the other foot.* | |

*(laughter)*

| SURGEON B | SURGEON A | SURGEON M |
|---|---|---|
| *Is this a...* | | *Why have they done this?* |
| | *Metatarsal amputation.* | |
| *The toes don't look so bad that...* | *No.* | *That one toe's a little, I don't know, is it arteriosclerosis obliterans or...* |
| | *Is there something in the sole of foot that we aren't seeing?* | *Yes, but quite, somehow it looks too good from this side for arteriosclerosis obliterans. Those wouldn't even bleed that much, would they?* |
| | *No, they wouldn't. Why have they left so much of that dermis, I mean, dorsal skin?* | *Indeed. Could this one be a tumor also?* |
| *Yeah.* | *Maybe.* | |
| *Diabetes related amputation. But it doesn't look like it.* | *It doesn't look like a diabetic...* | *But the diabetic doesn't need to have arteriosclerosis obliterans. If it's neuropathic and there are awful wounds there on the sole...* |
| | *Yes, there's some...* | |
| *In the ball of the foot...* | *...dent in the ball of the foot.* | |
| *It's like...* | *It is in a way, adorable that big toe and the little ones; it's a sort of little guy.* | |
| *Here you can see, like, your own development in these amputation procedures. I remember when I was quite new in the business, I thought it was very dramatic and I think the patients also took it quite hard. Now it's more like routine. Just snip away a toe and it doesn't make such an impression anymore.* | *This is a nice one.* | *I'm still wondering that... Okay, diabetes, but why did they end up doing this?* |
| | *I don't quite get it either. Why take so much off the foot?* | |
| *The ball of the foot must have...* | | *But wouldn't for example the Charcot foot... And even if there were ulcers, there are all sorts of medical shoes and...* |
| | *Indeed, and casts and...* | *And then you can kind of ossify the foot and...* |
| | *But could there still be some osteomyelitis somewhere over there...* | *That we just aren't seeing.* |

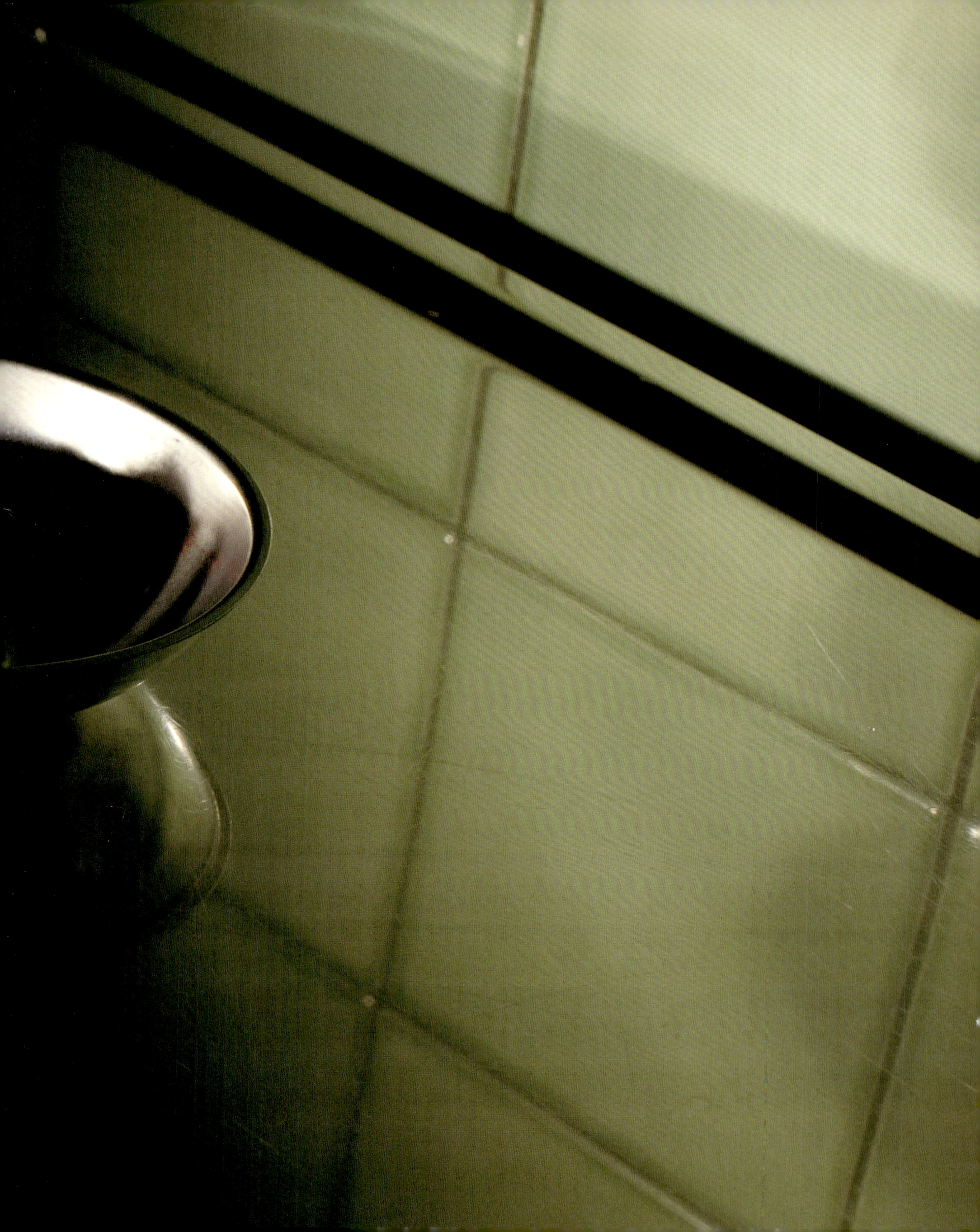

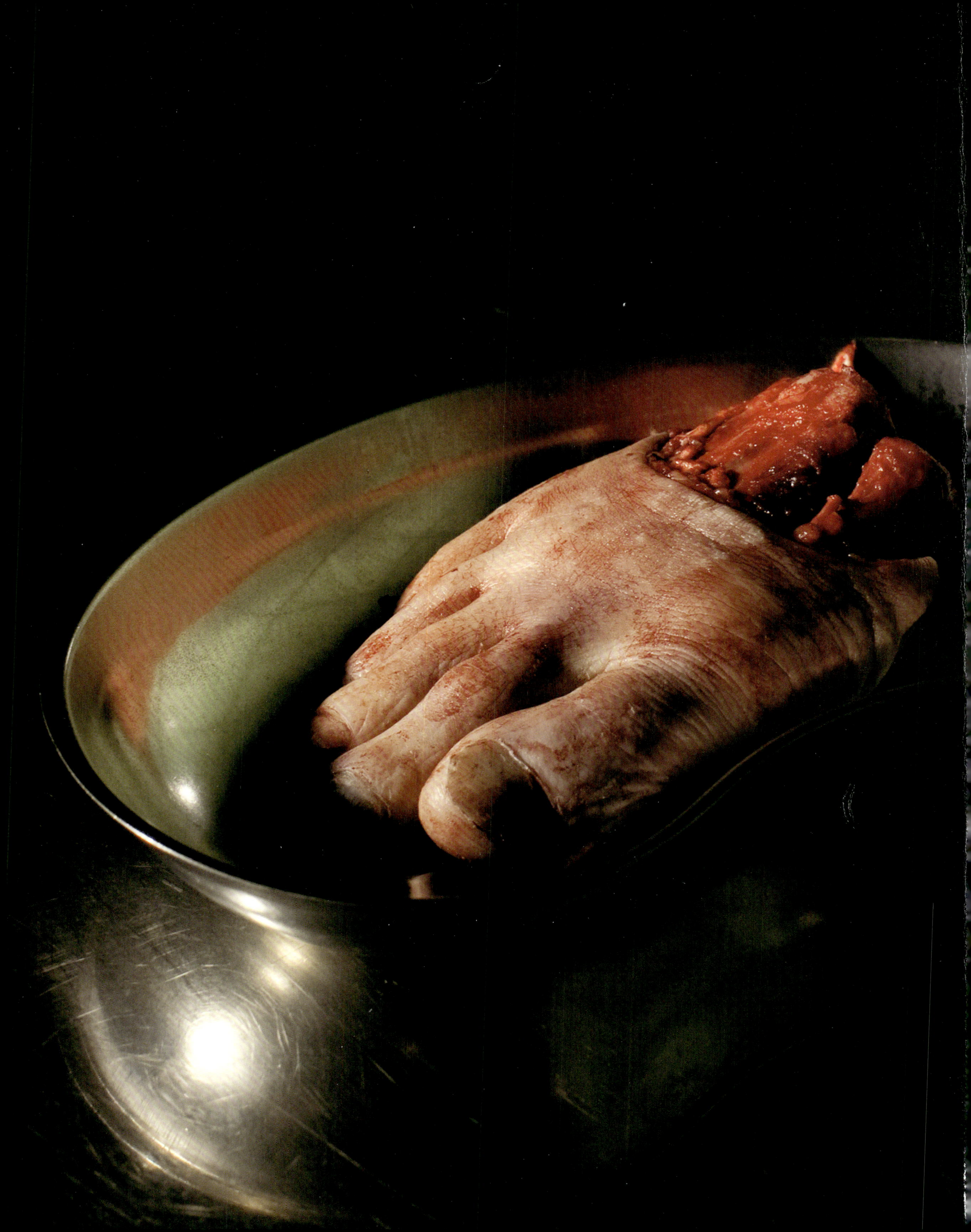

MAIJA TAMMI is a photographer, artist and researcher. She is currently working on her doctoral thesis on representations of sickness in art photography at Aalto University's Doctoral Programme in Arts, Design and Architecture in Helsinki, Finland.

Book design by
VILLE TIETÄVÄINEN
/Studio Tietäväinen Oy

Discussants are three surgeons in Finland:
ANTTI MIKKOLA specializes in plastic surgery,
BERENT MUNSTERHJELM in general surgery, and
MAINA JALAVA in orthopaedics.
Translation from Finnish to English by
MINNA SAARI



Printed in Germany

ISBN 978-3-86828-522-2

Kehrer Heidelberg Berlin
www.kehrerverlag.com

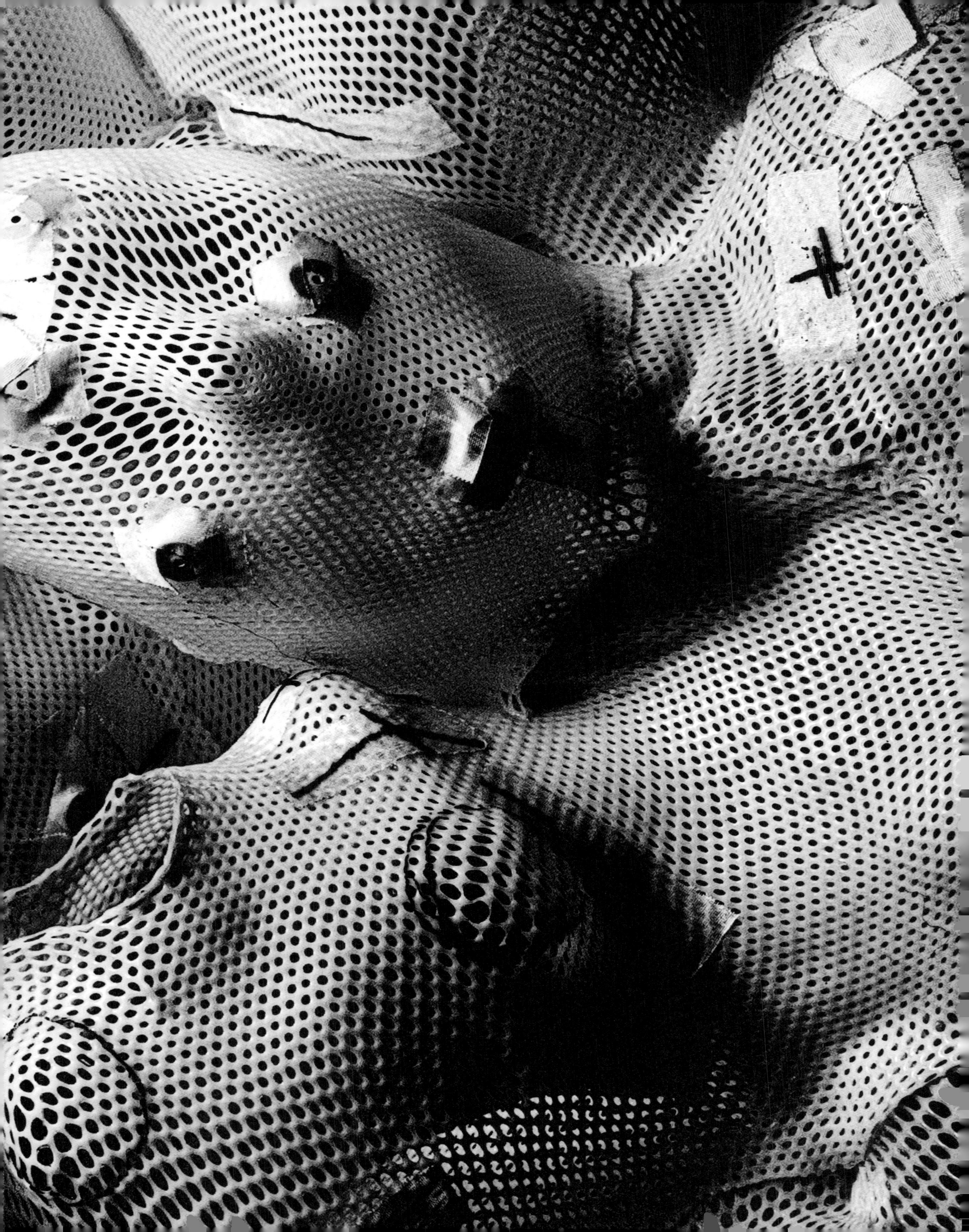

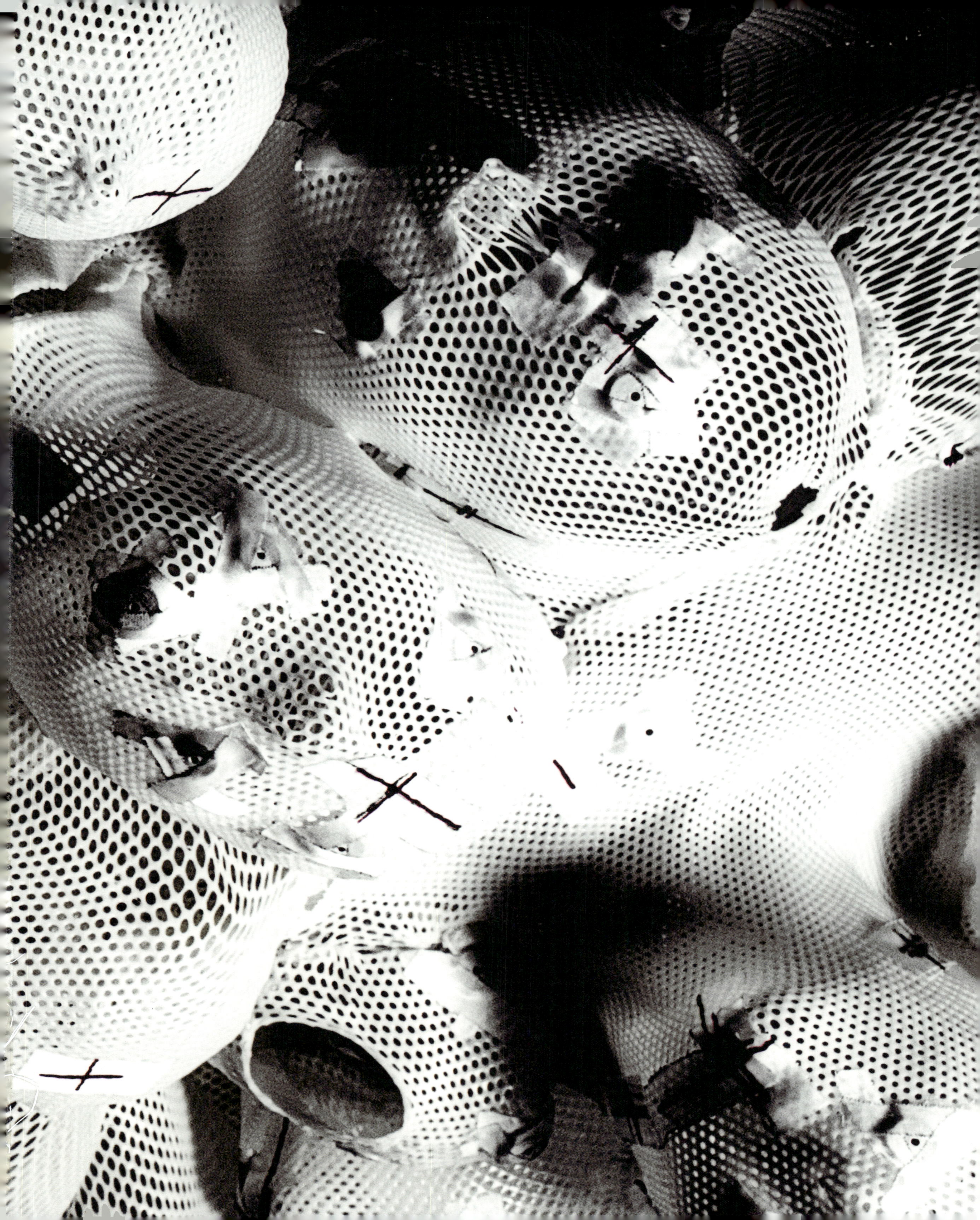

# LEFTOVER

Used radiotherapy masks from Helsinki University Central Hospital,
Turku University Hospital and Tampere University Hospital.

*That is what worries me.*

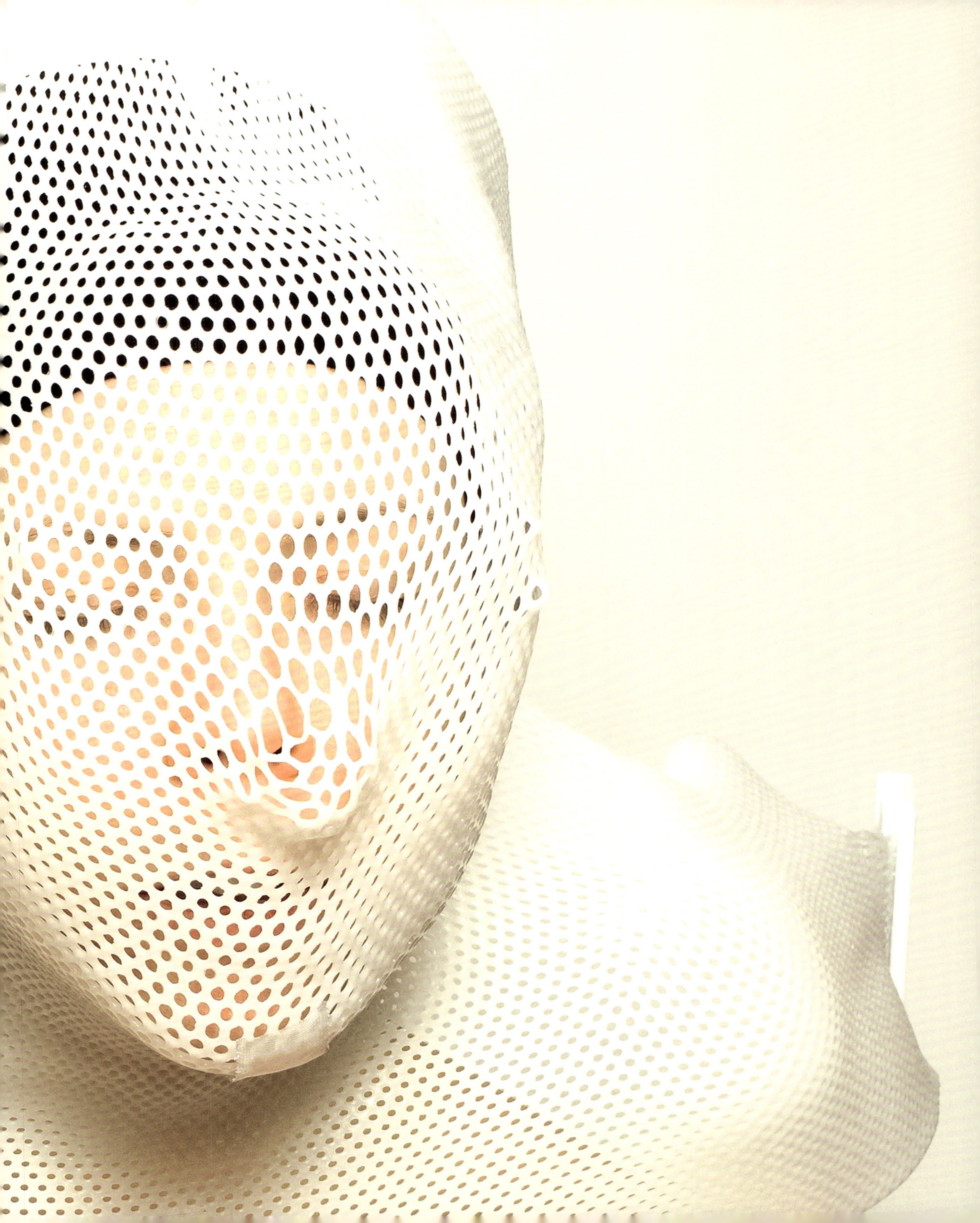

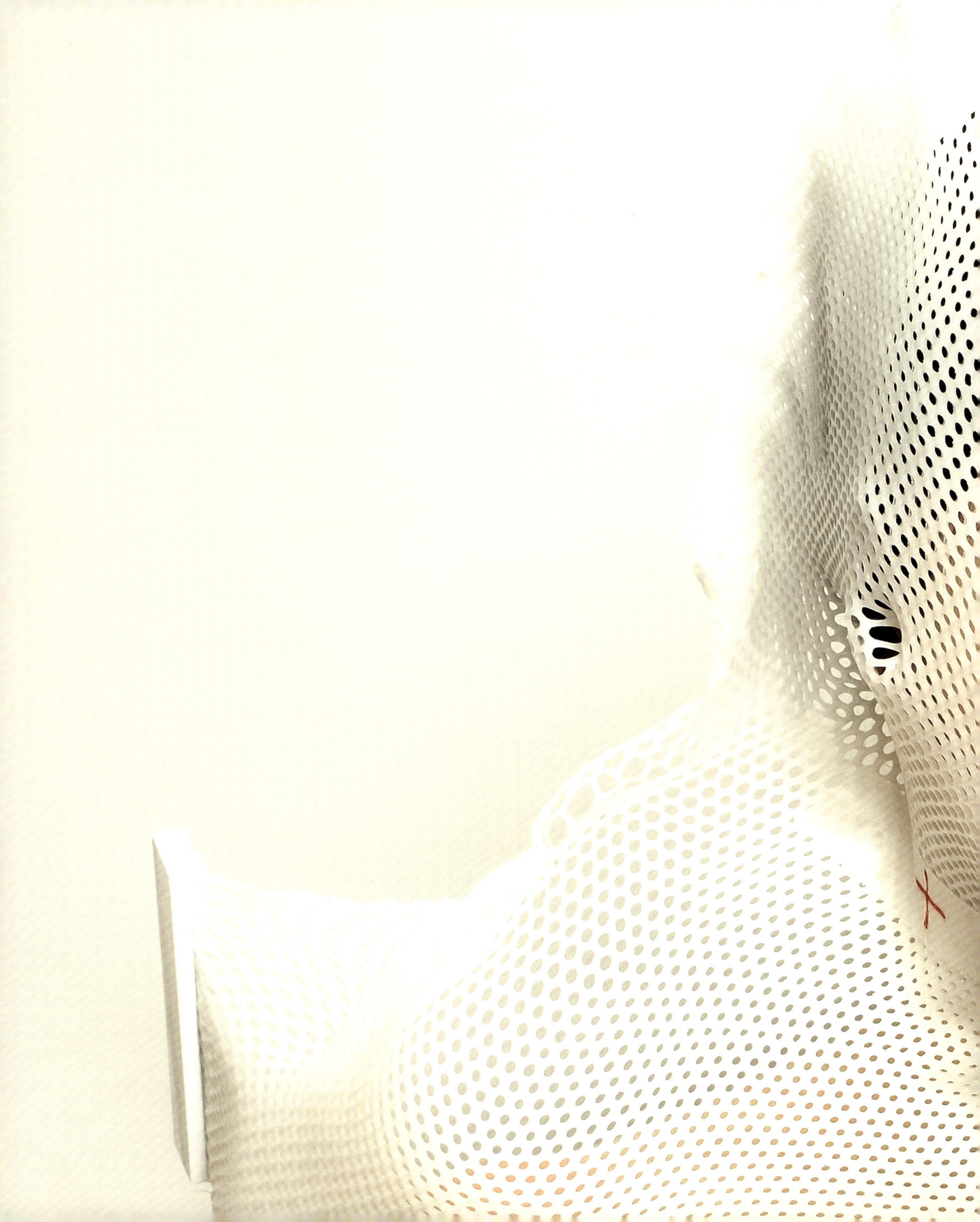

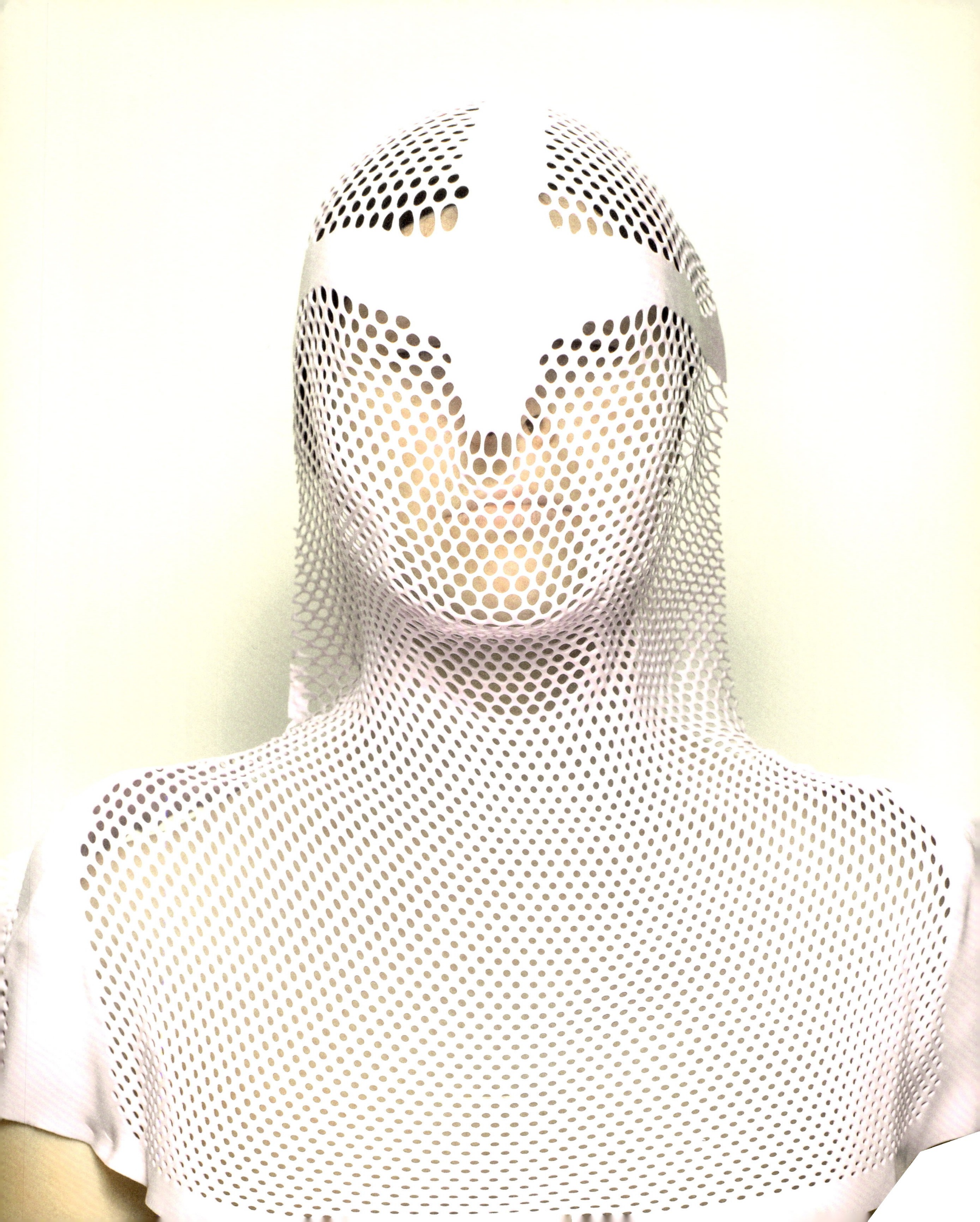

*I'll find you, don't worry about that.*

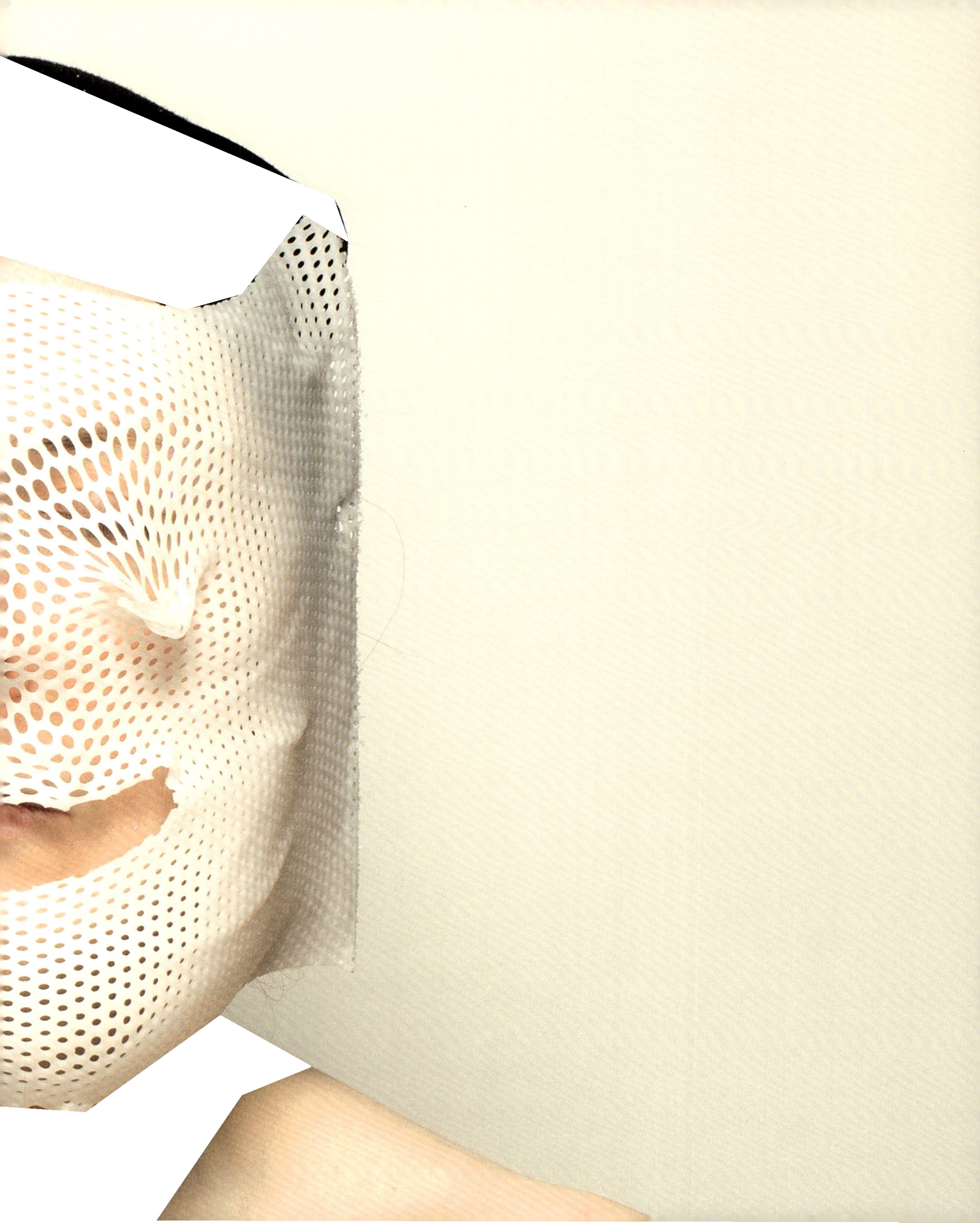

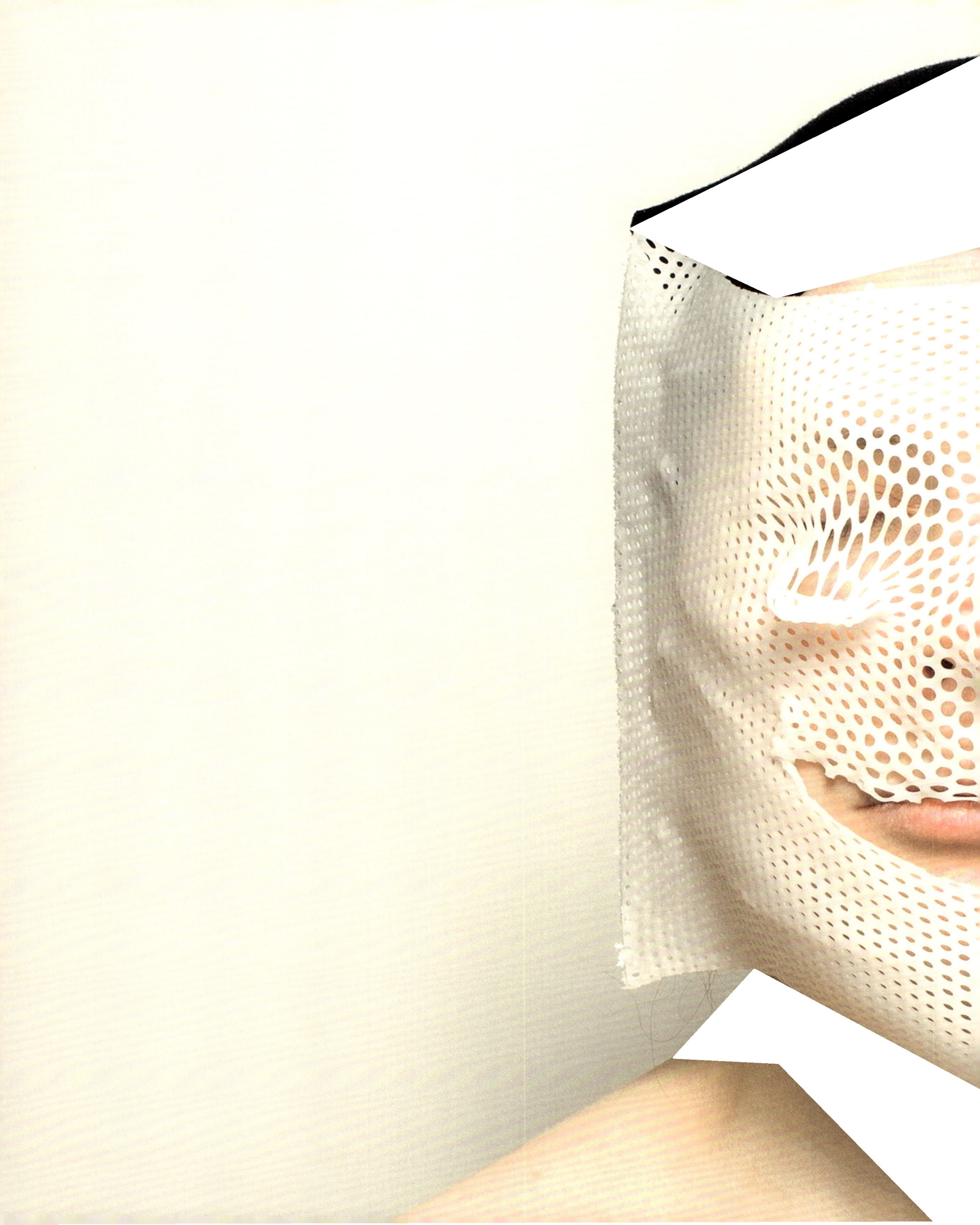

*How do I recognize you?*

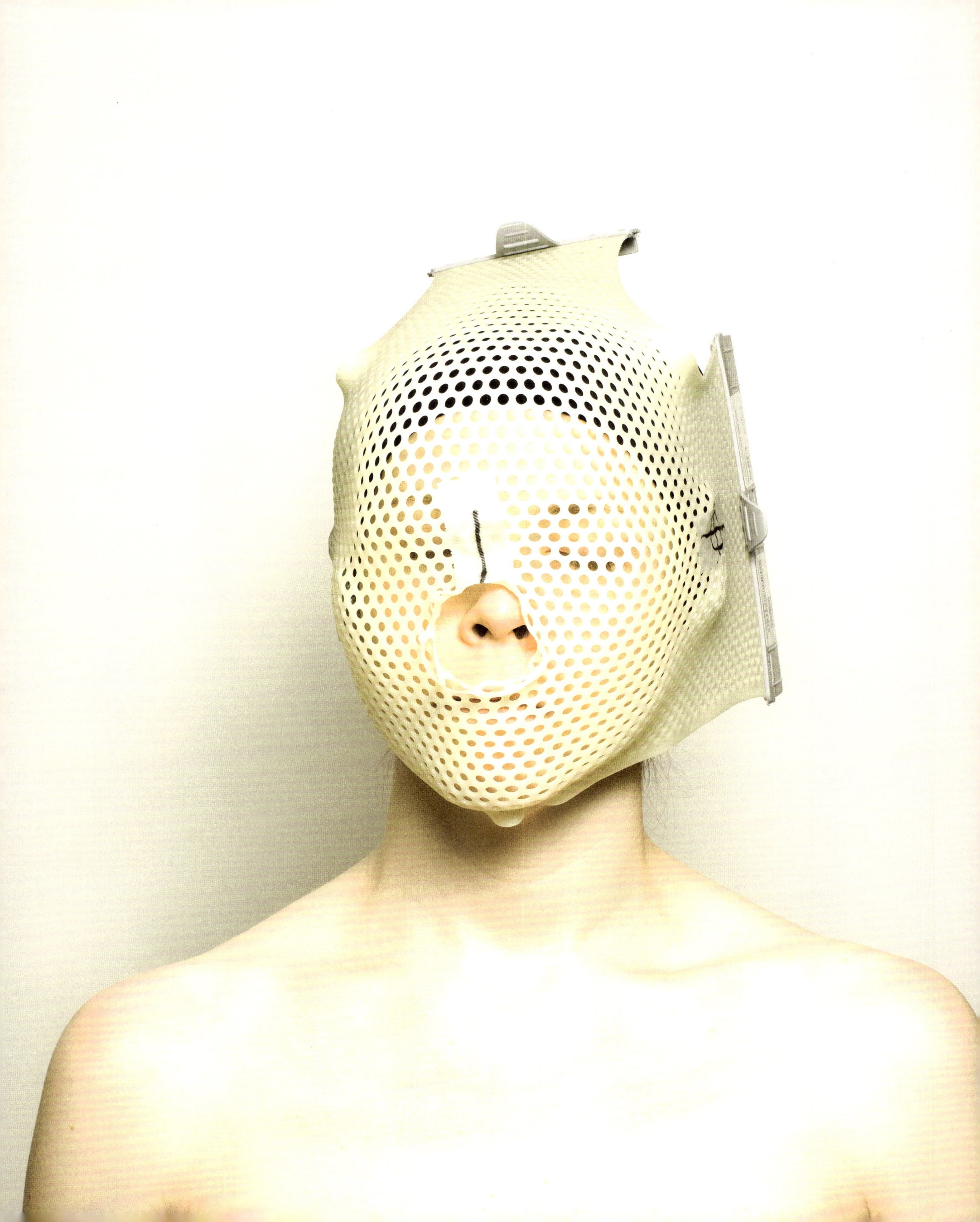

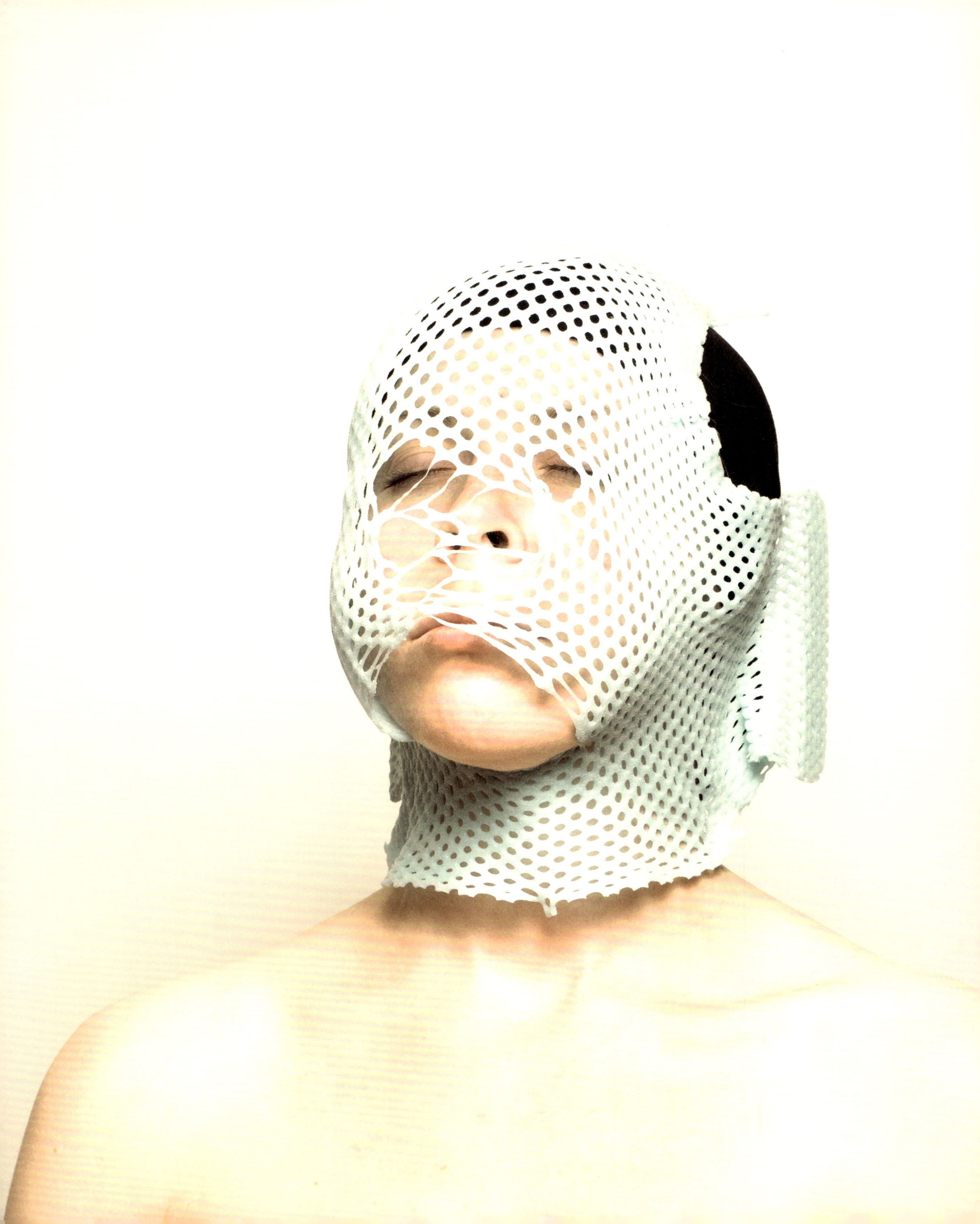

*I'll be right here.*

*Fine. Let's meet,* I SAY.
*Where do you want to meet?*
*Somewhere were you can smoke?*

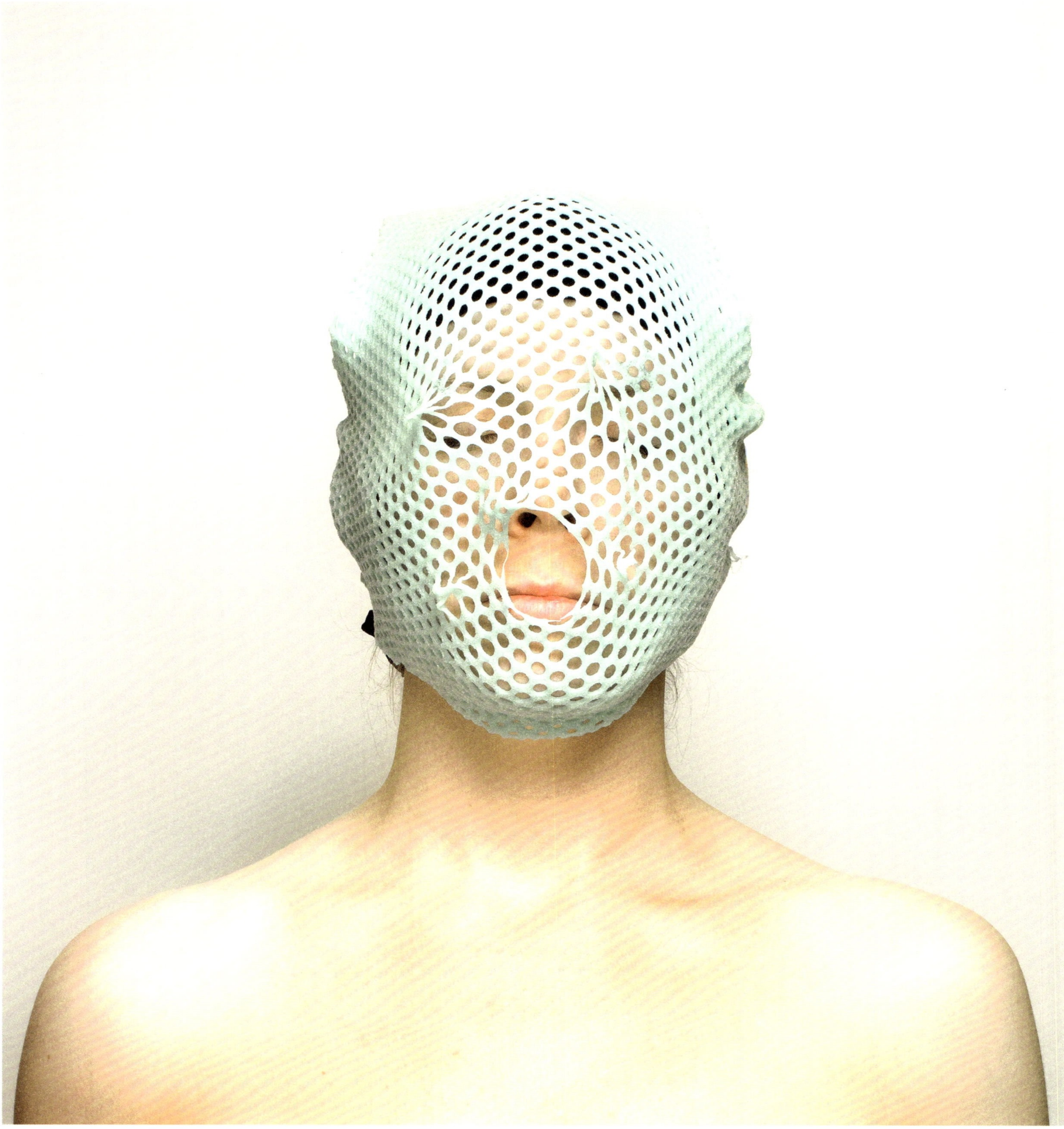

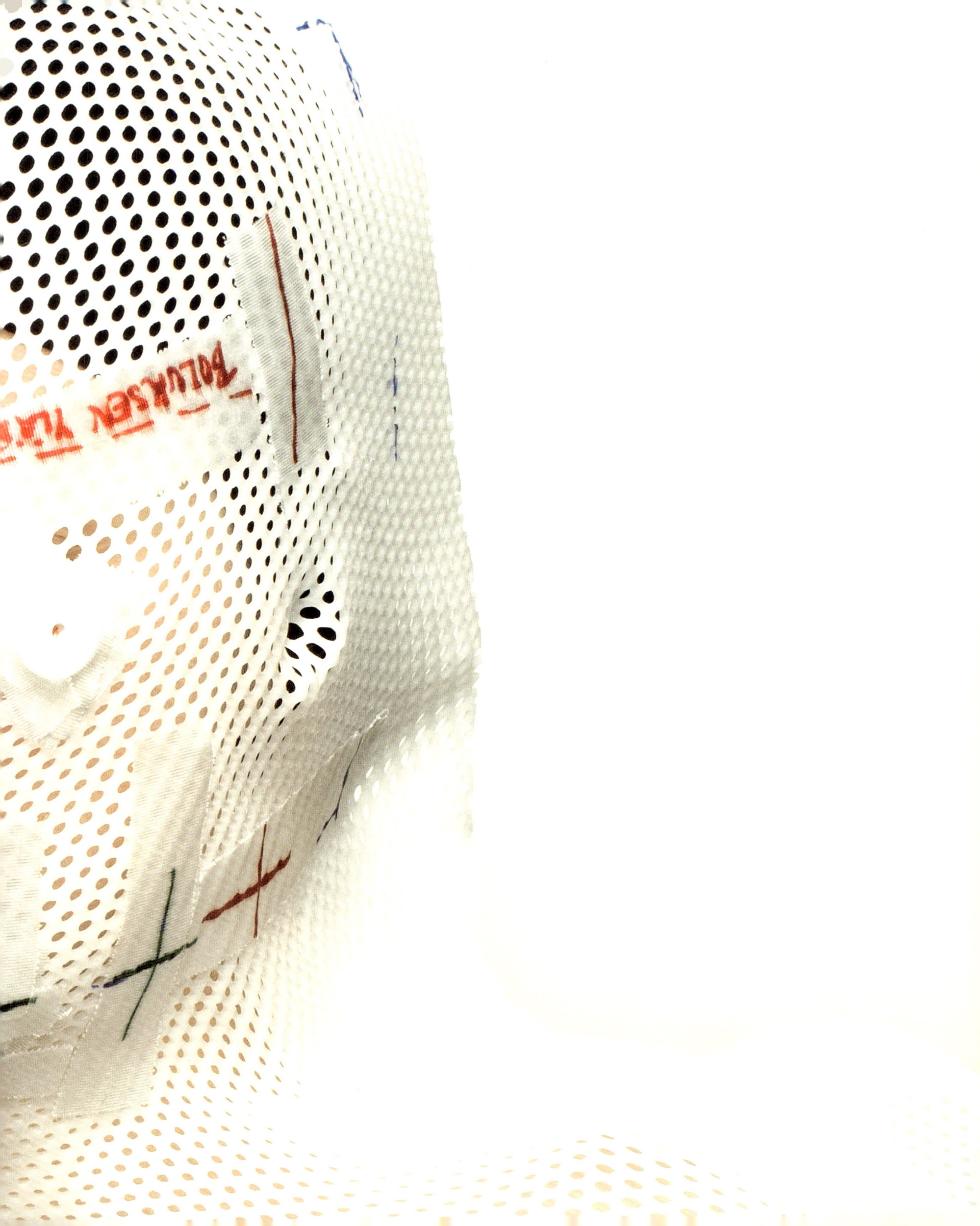

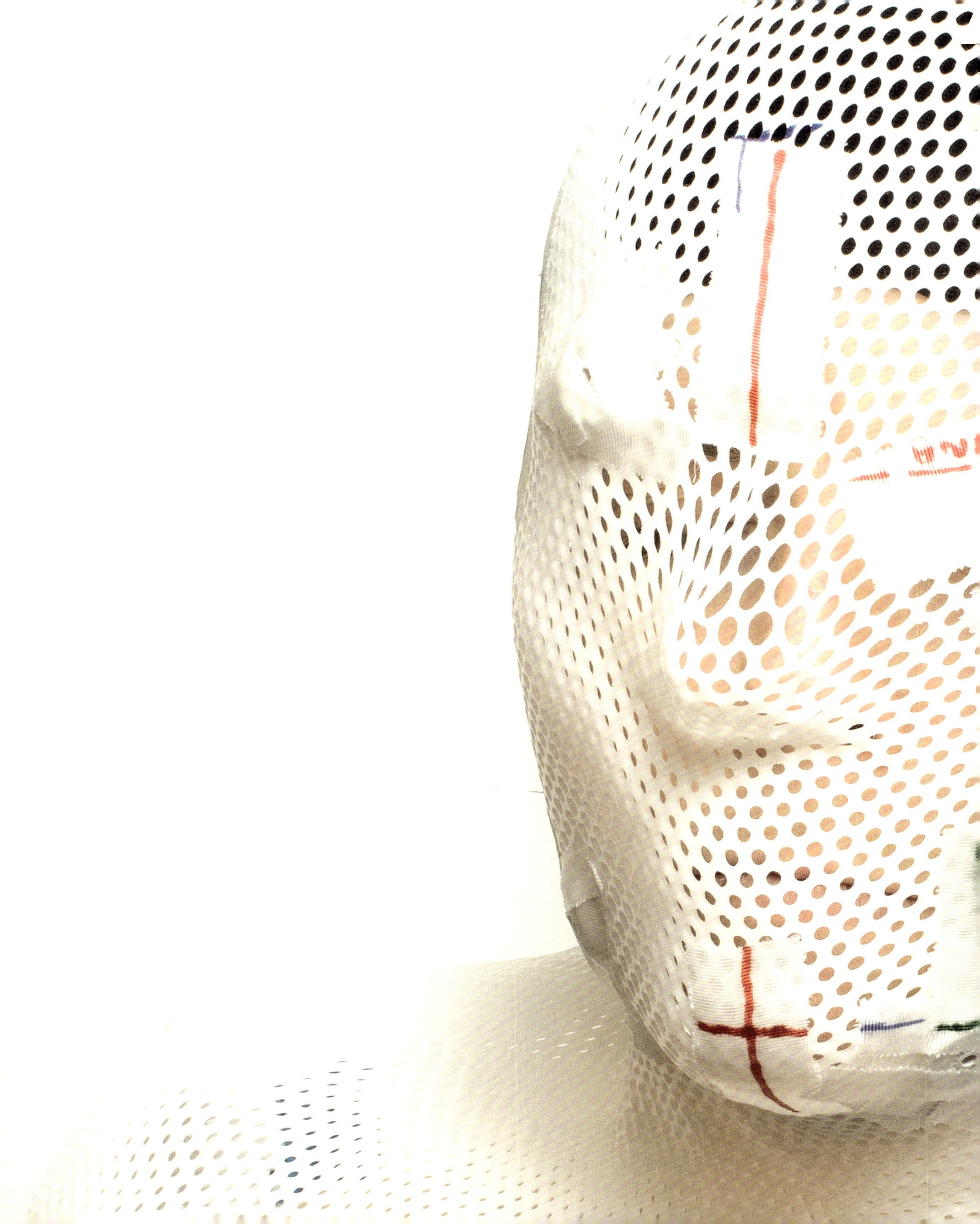

No reply.

*Yet,* I SAY. *Give me ten more years.*

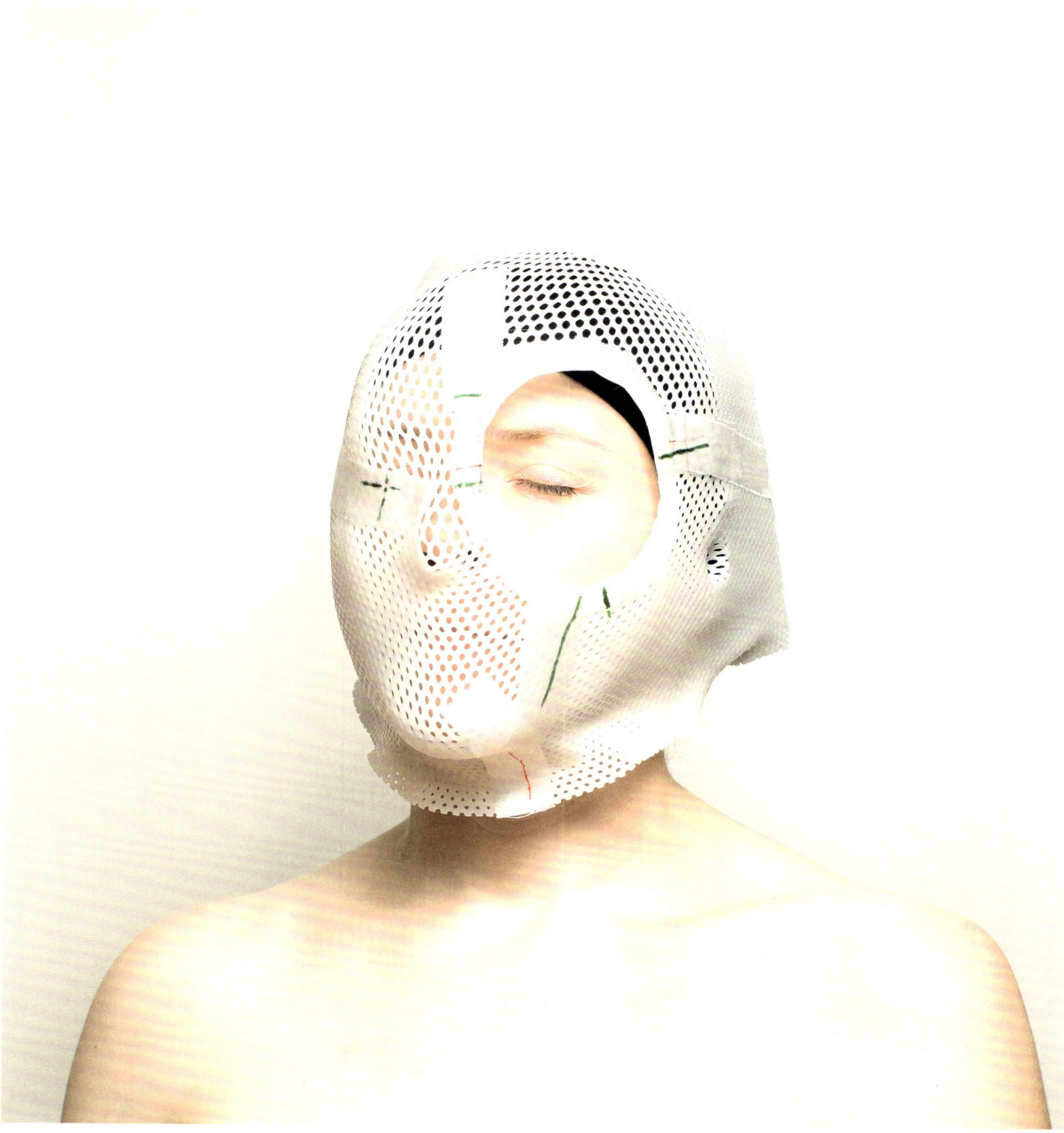

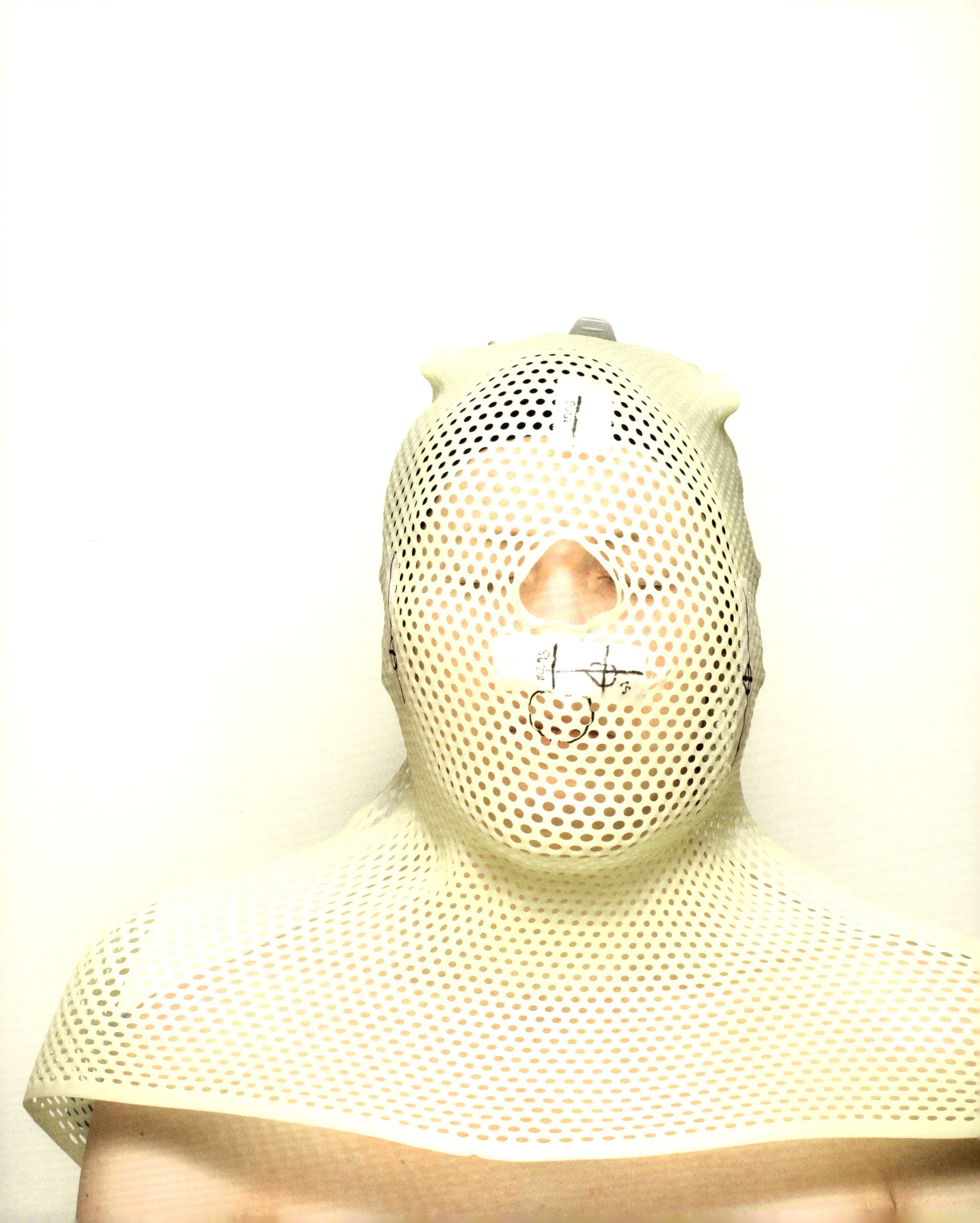

*Yet*, YOU SAY.

*I cannot feel you.*

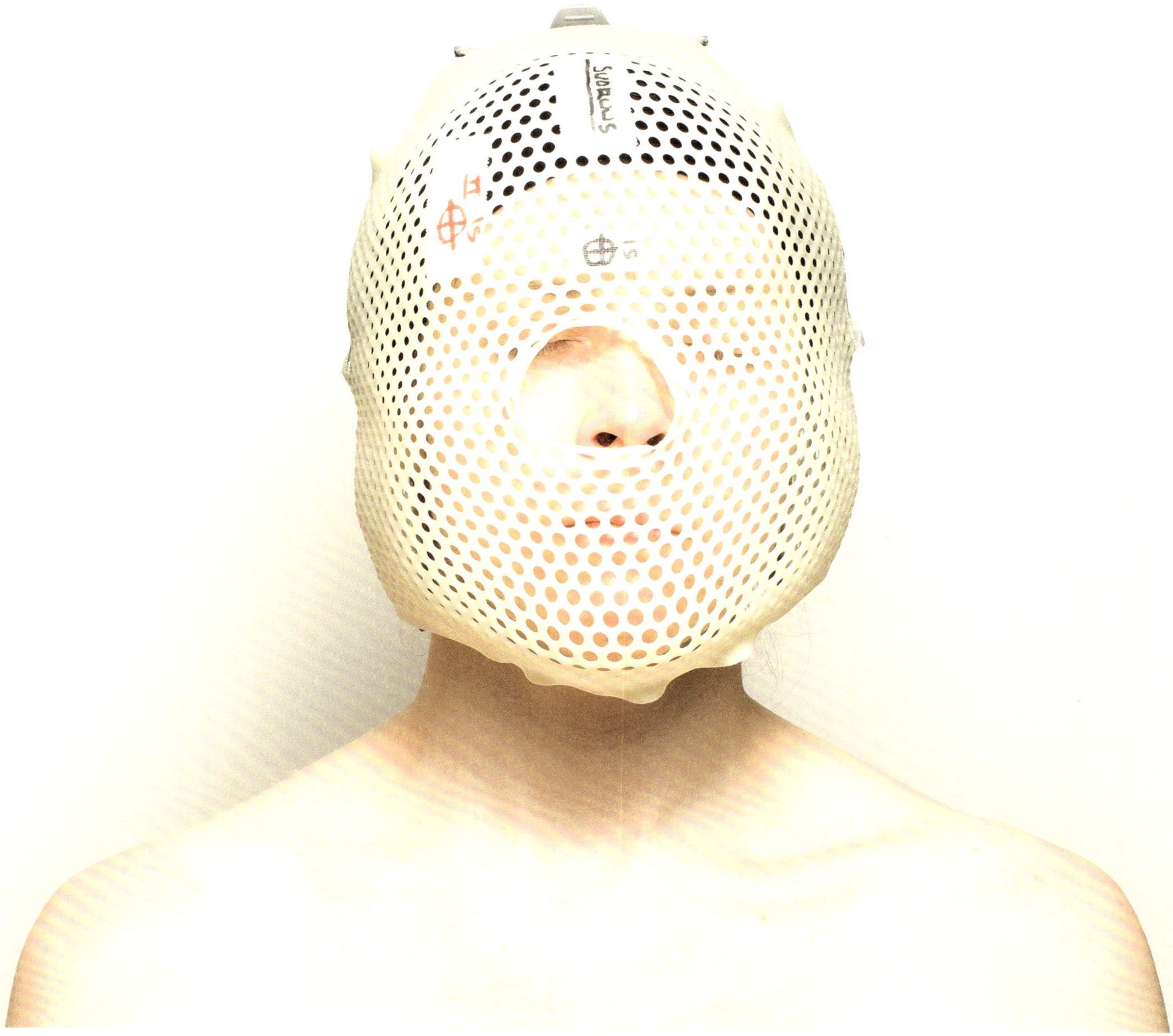

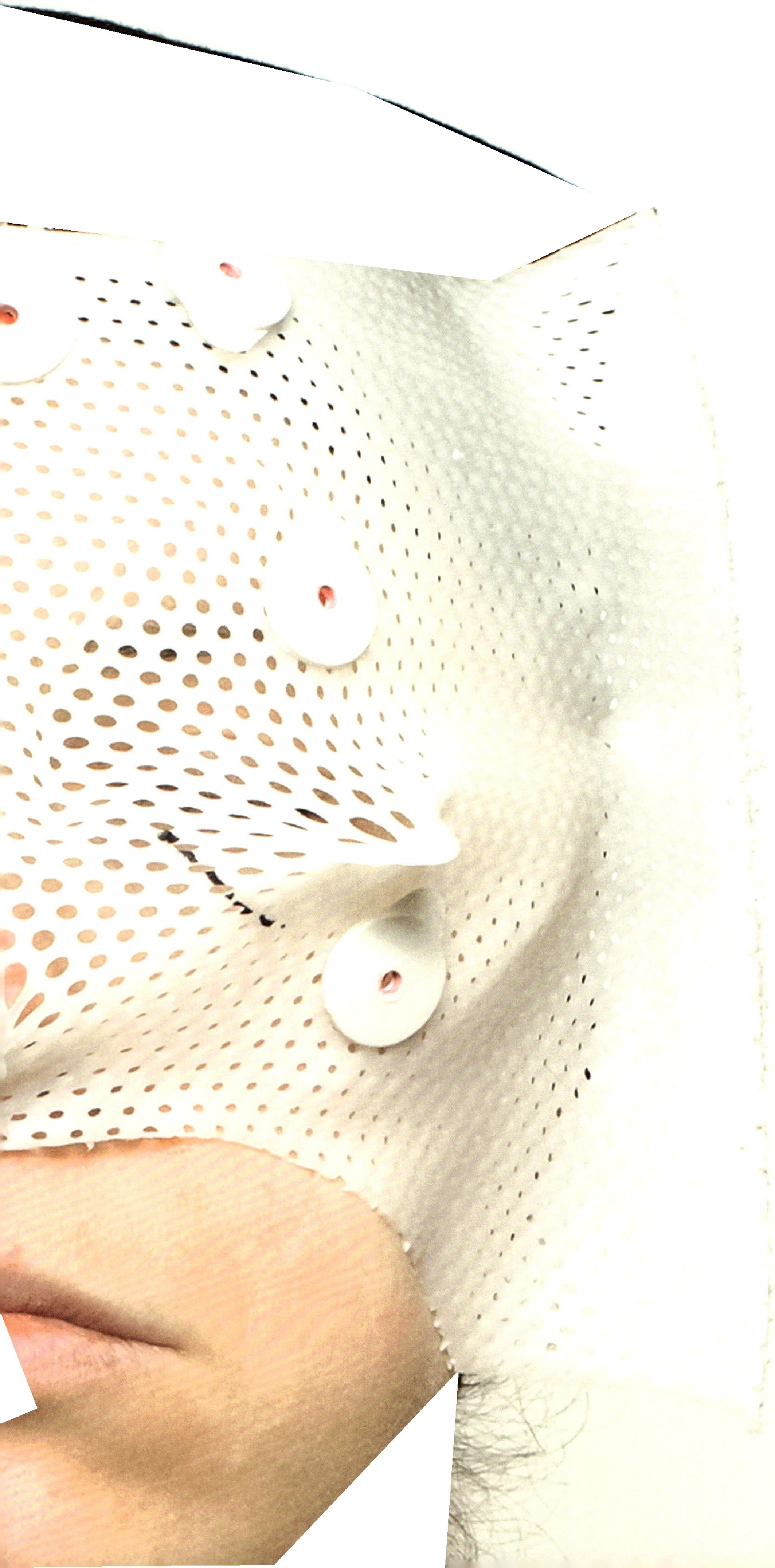

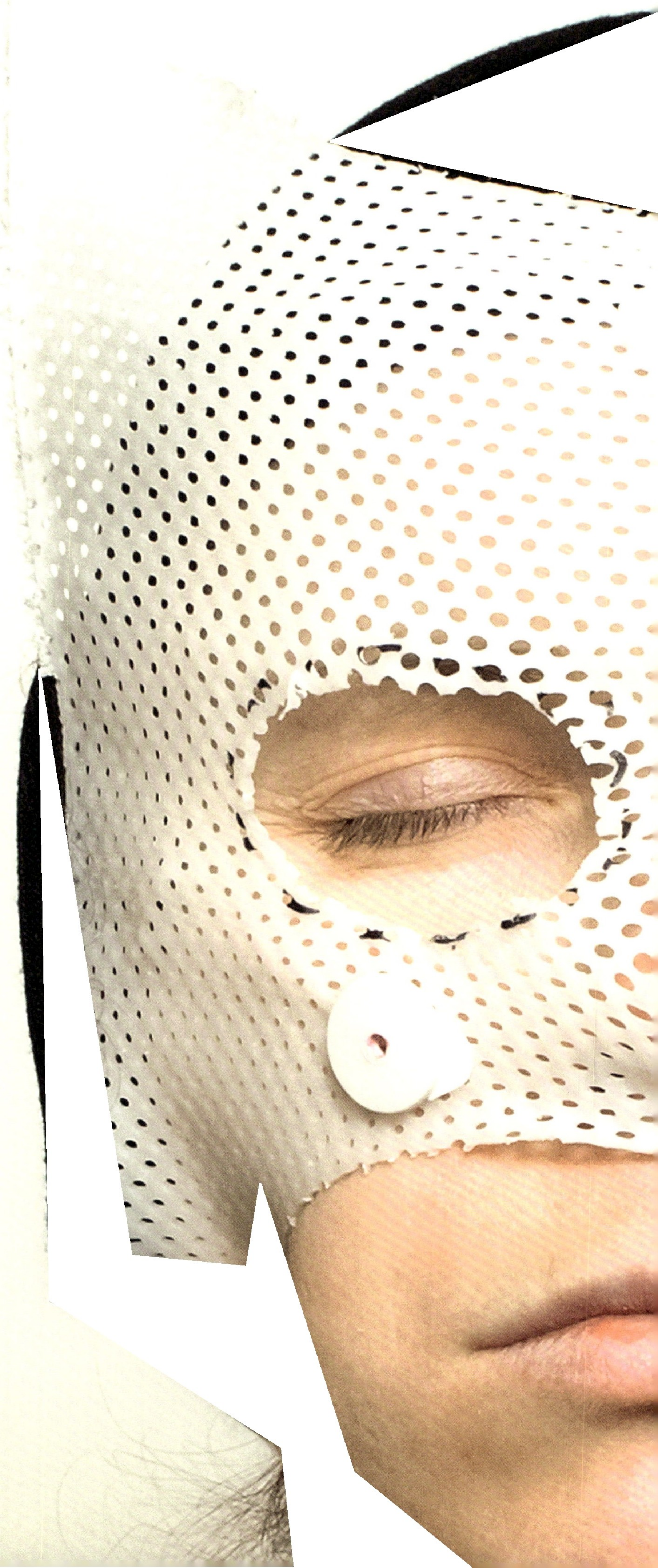

No answer.

*Are you trying to say that you are here now?*

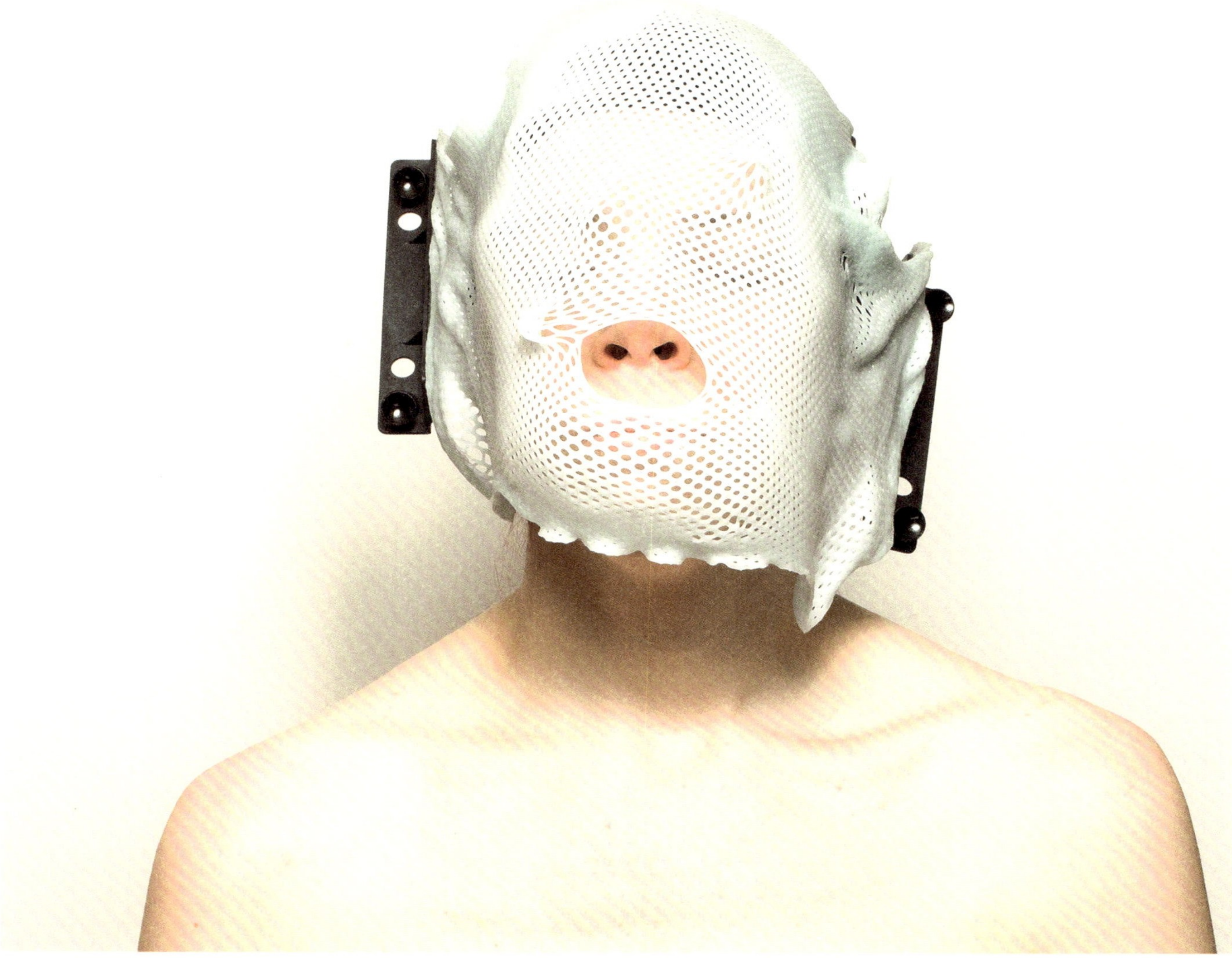

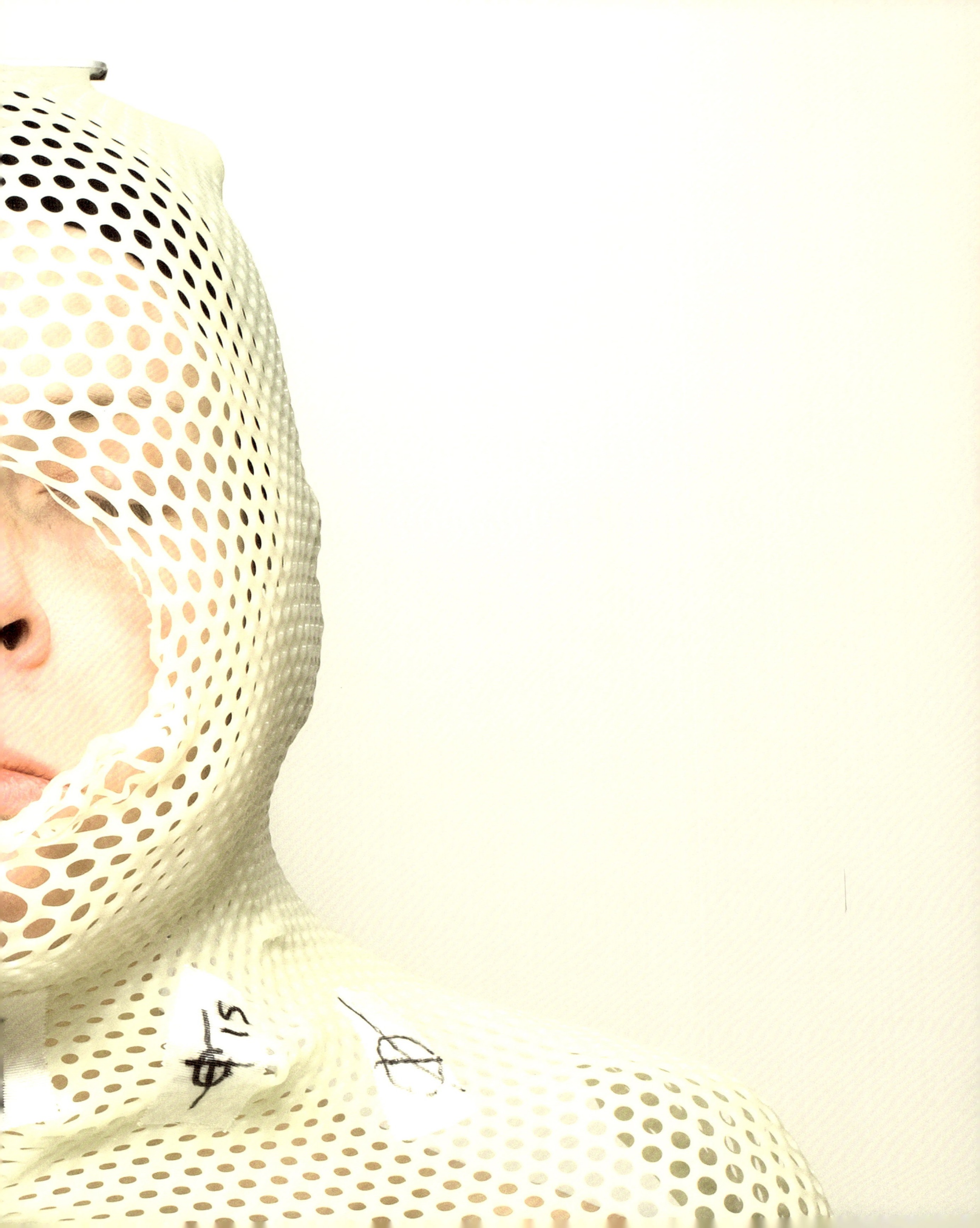
15

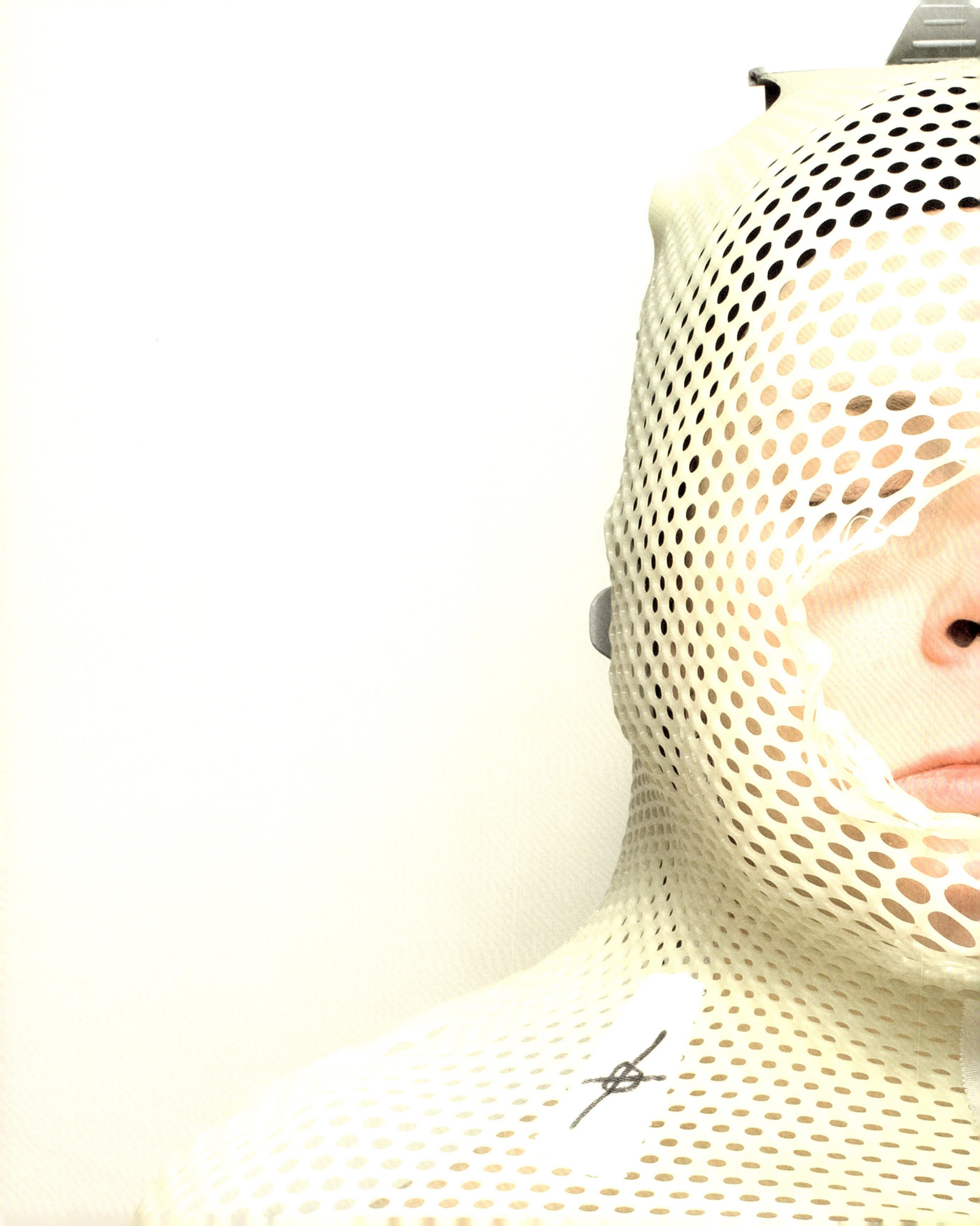

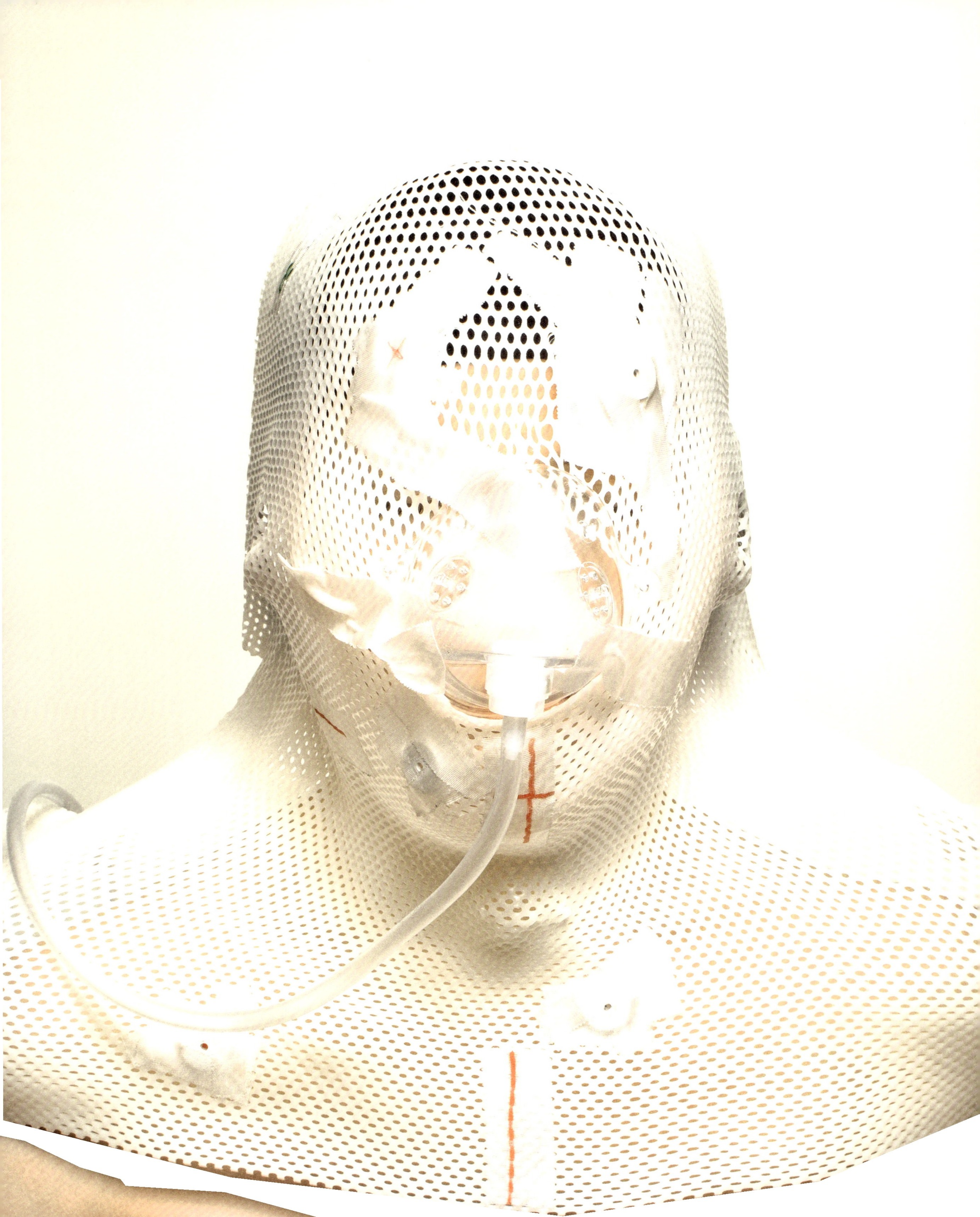

*I am part of life, brainless lump of your cells, part of you.*

*I don't know… life.*

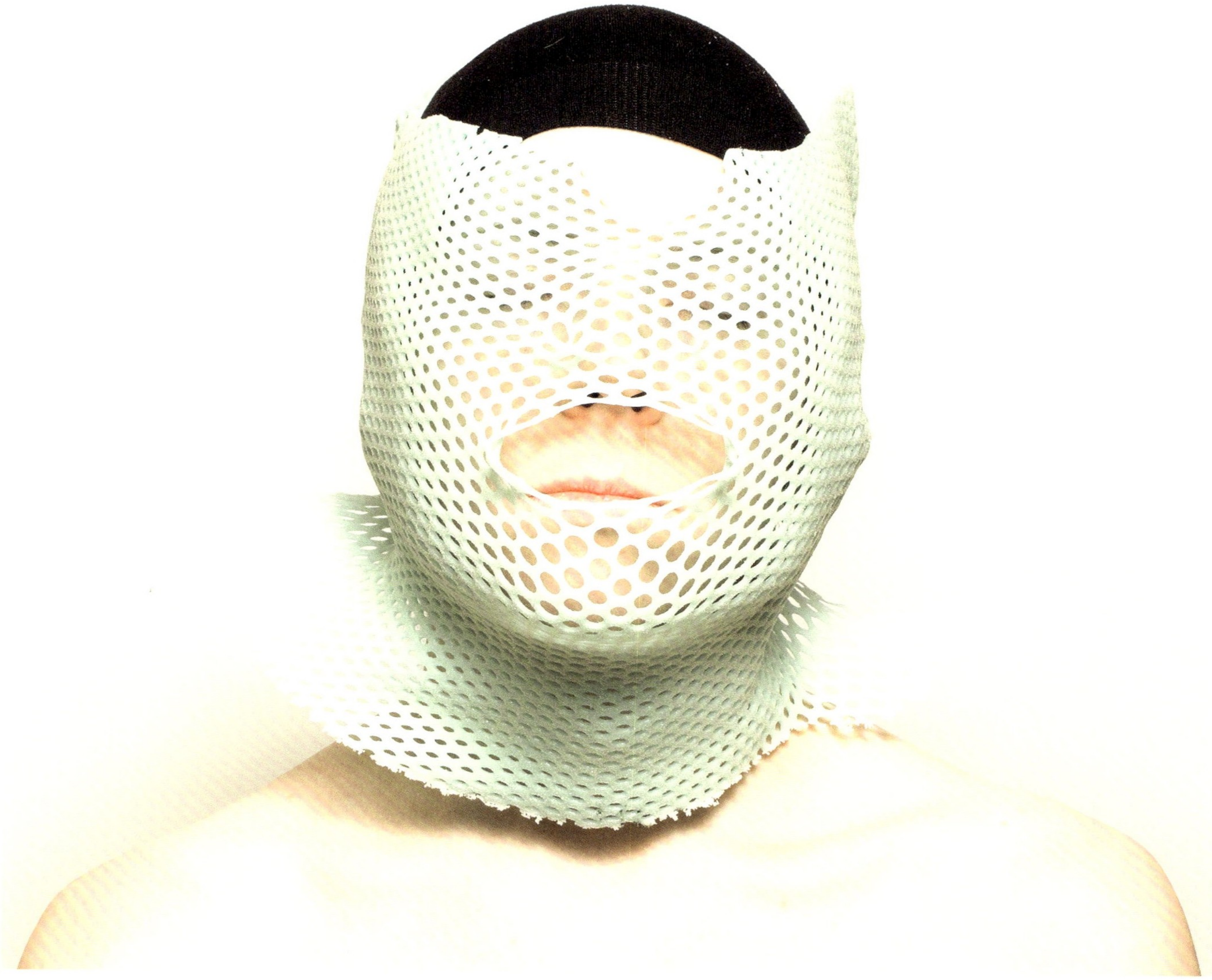

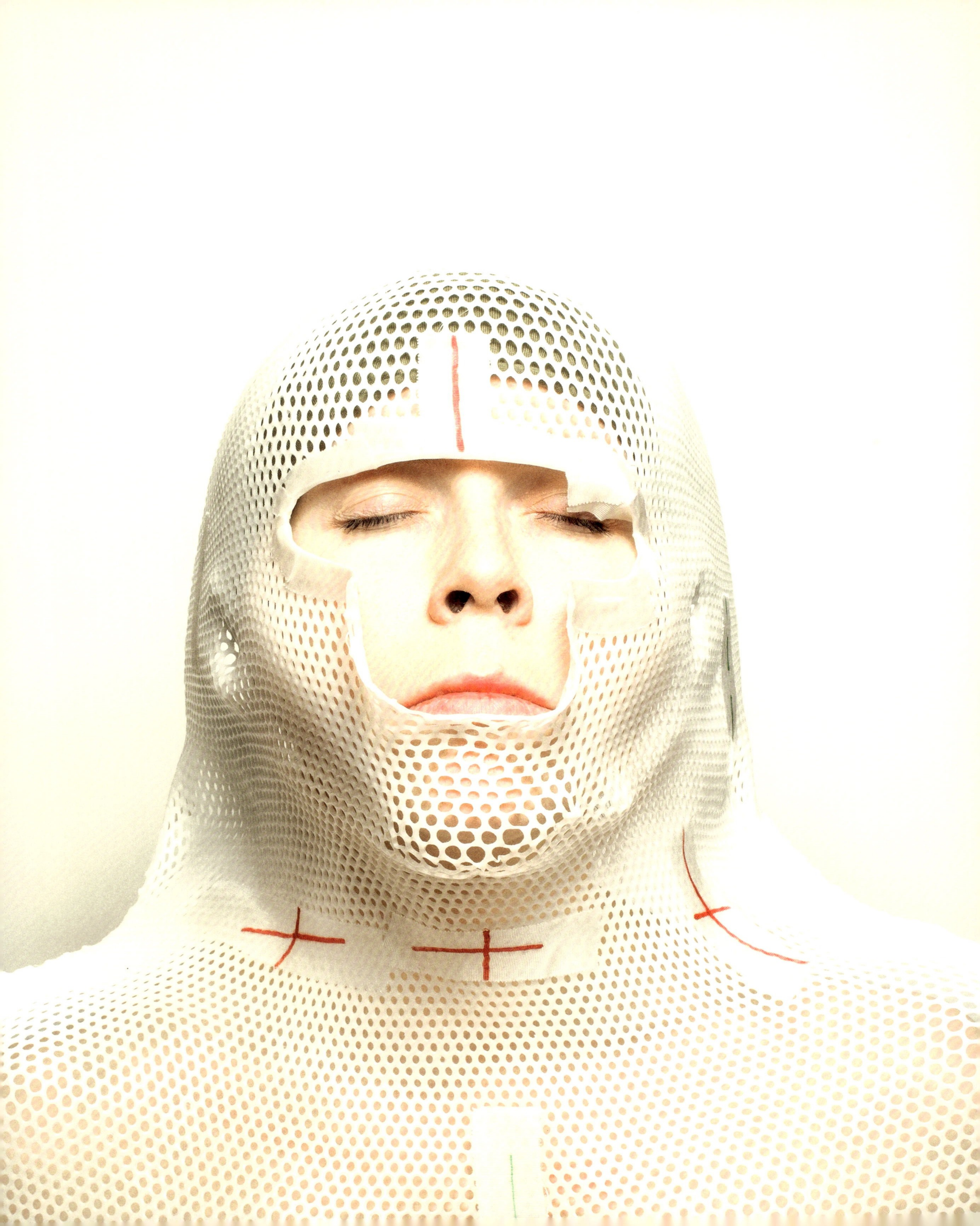

*What are you so busy with?*

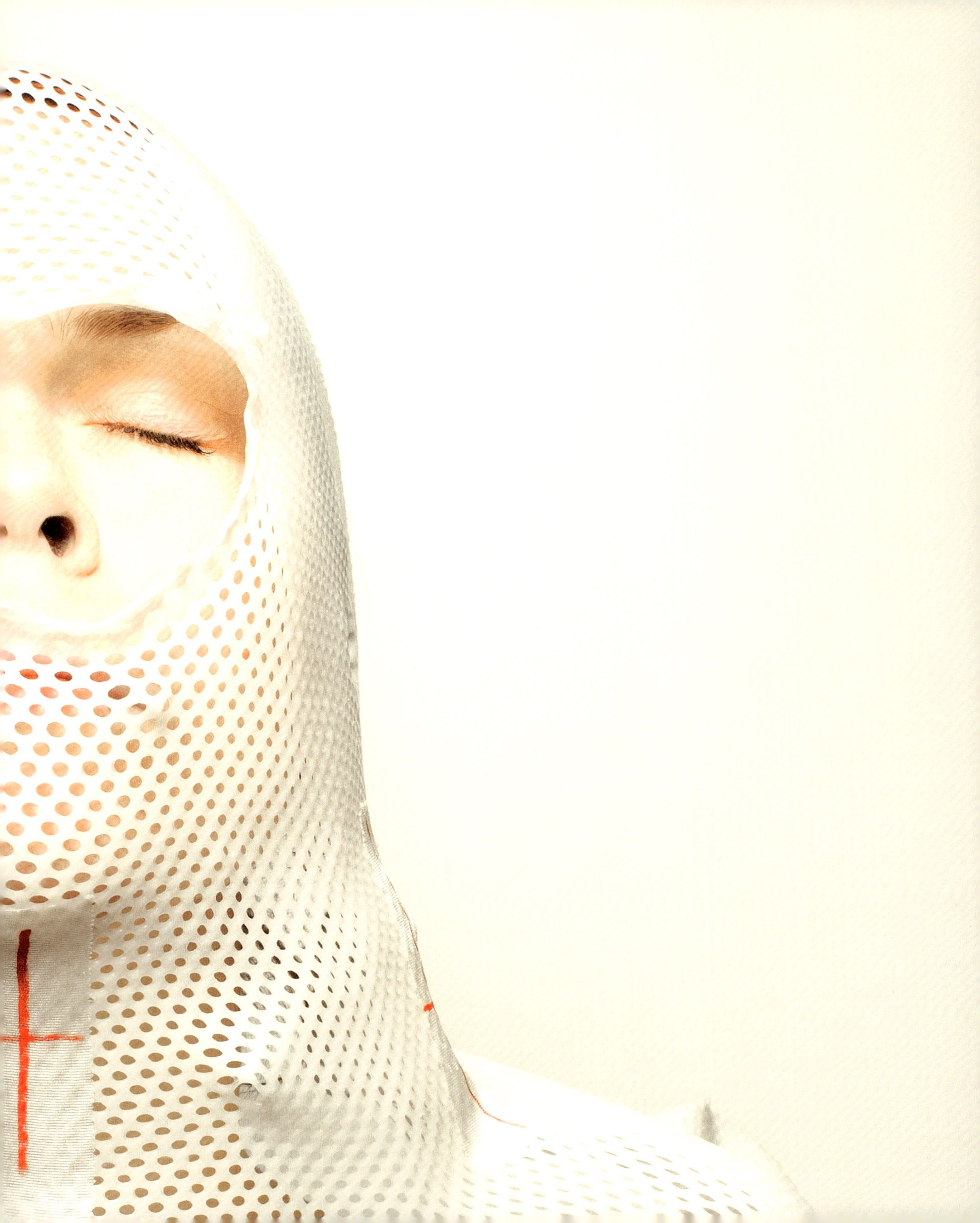

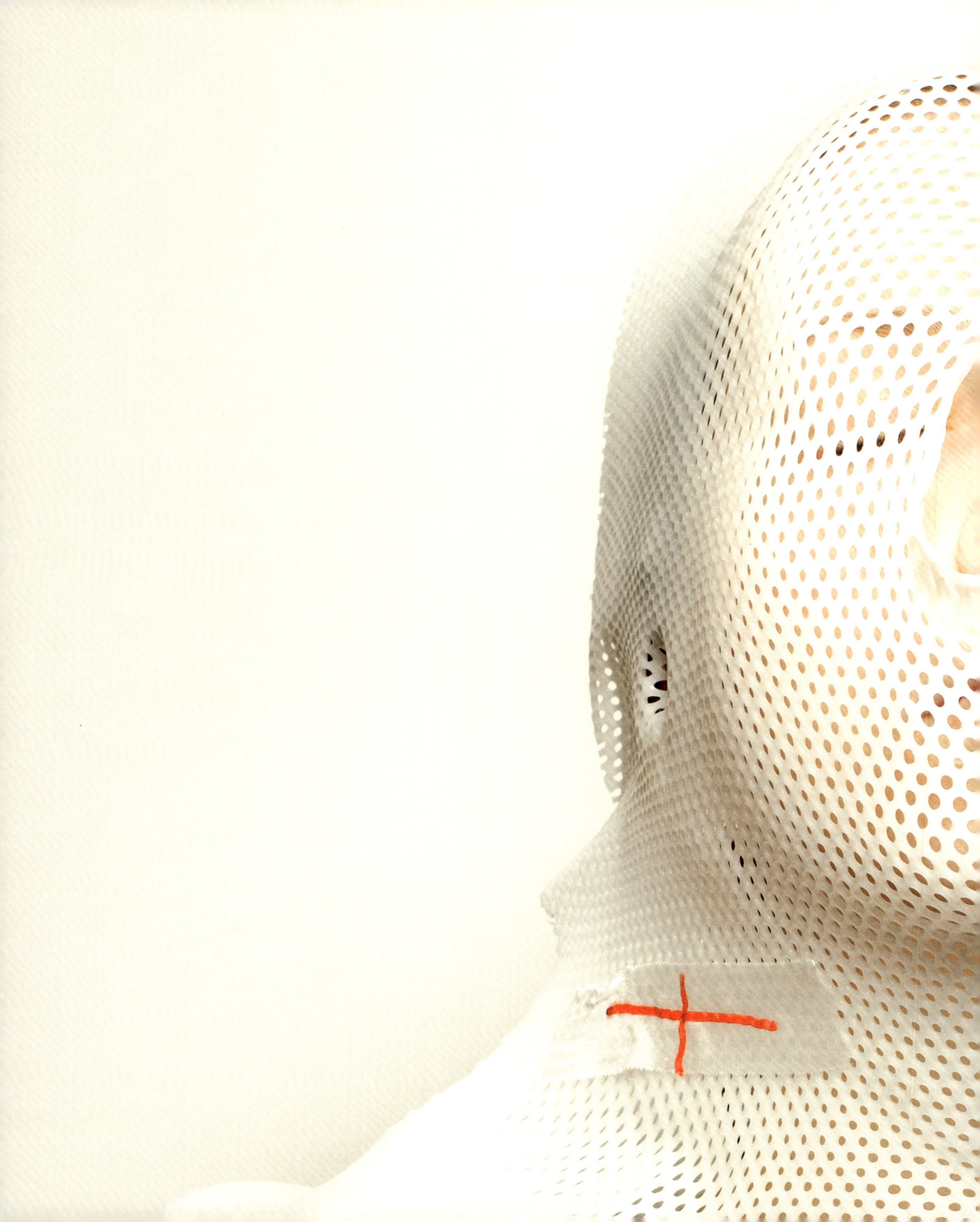

*I would rather meet you later then.*

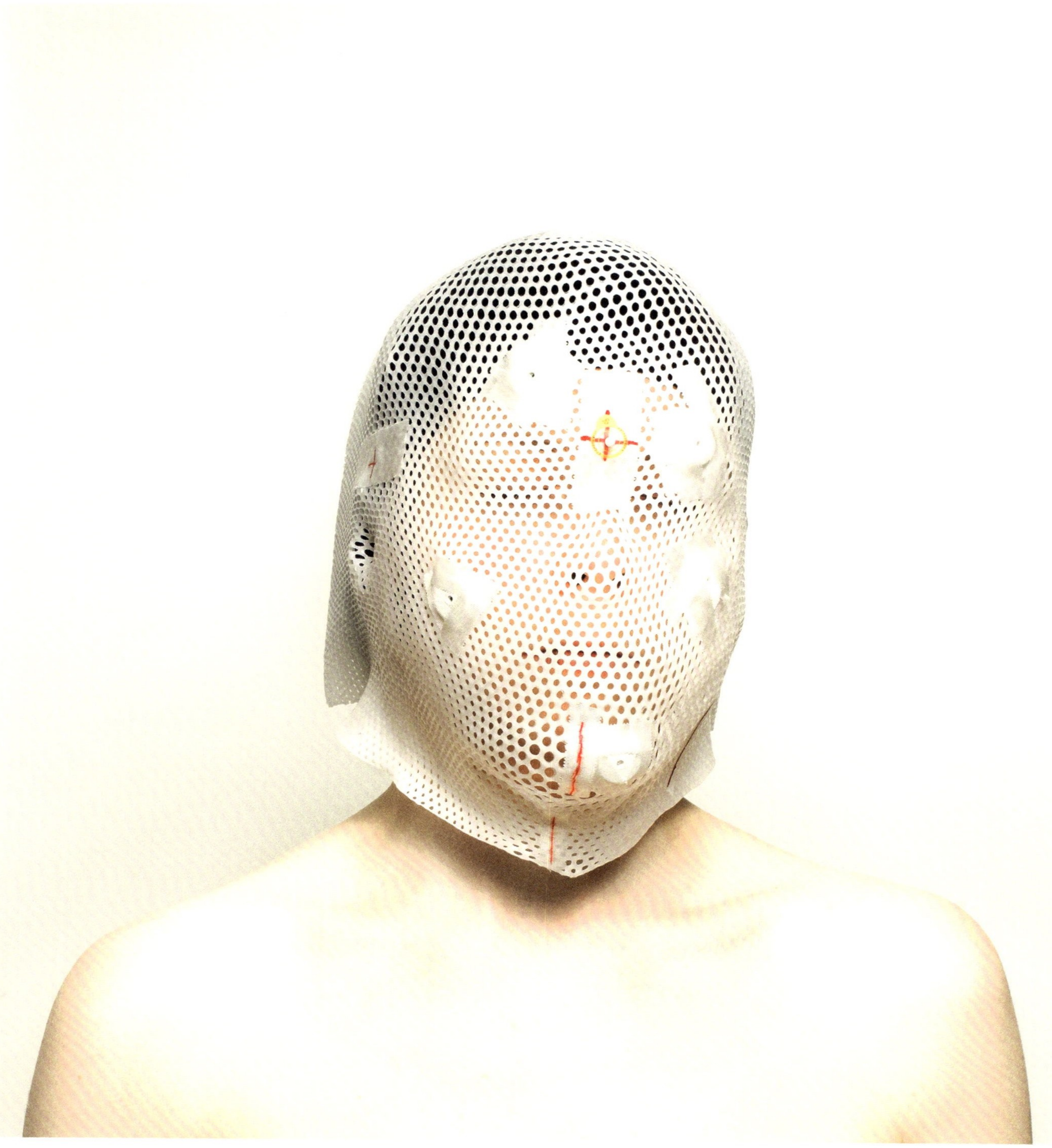

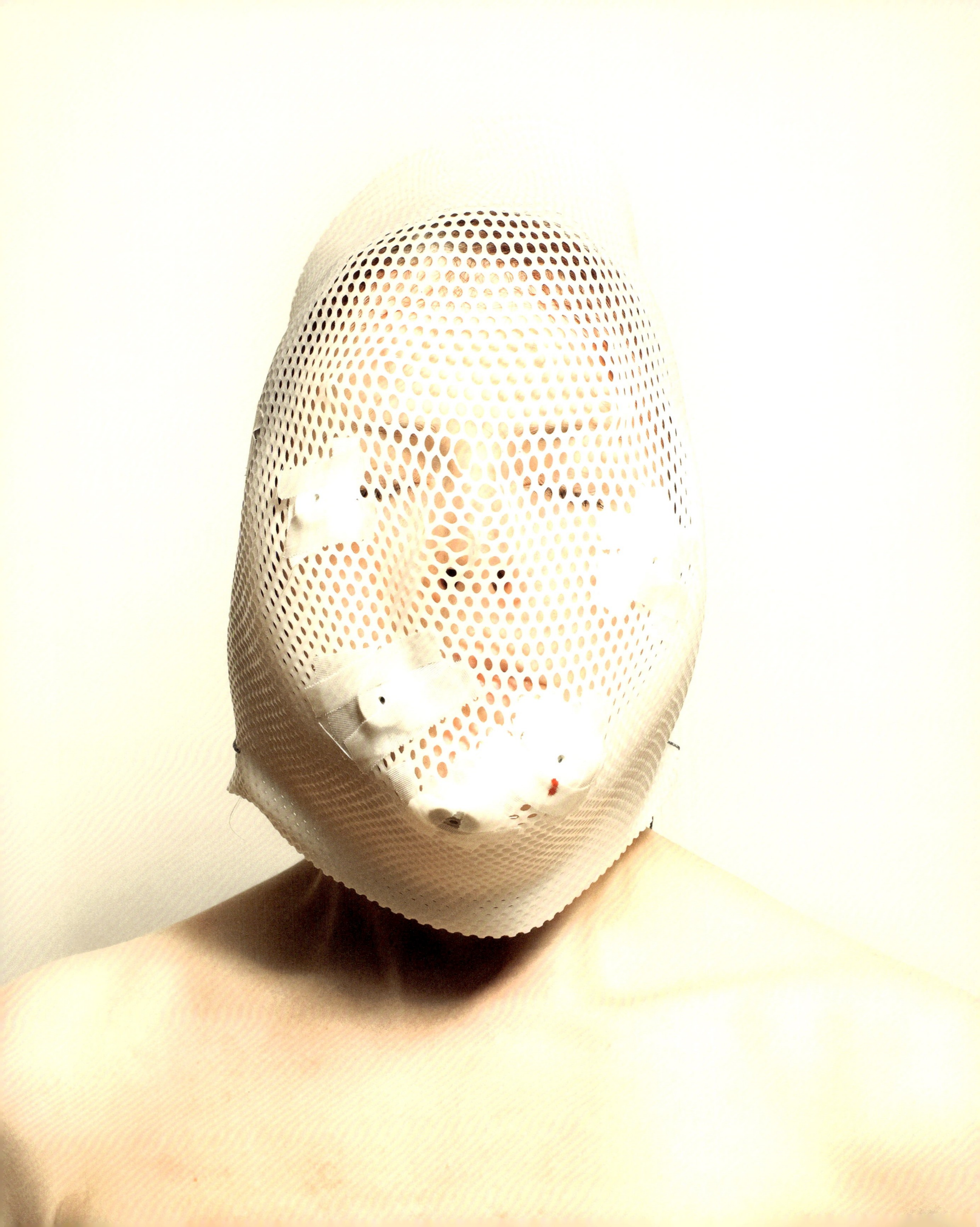

*I have time. I just multiply.*

*No! Thank you, I am busy with other things.*

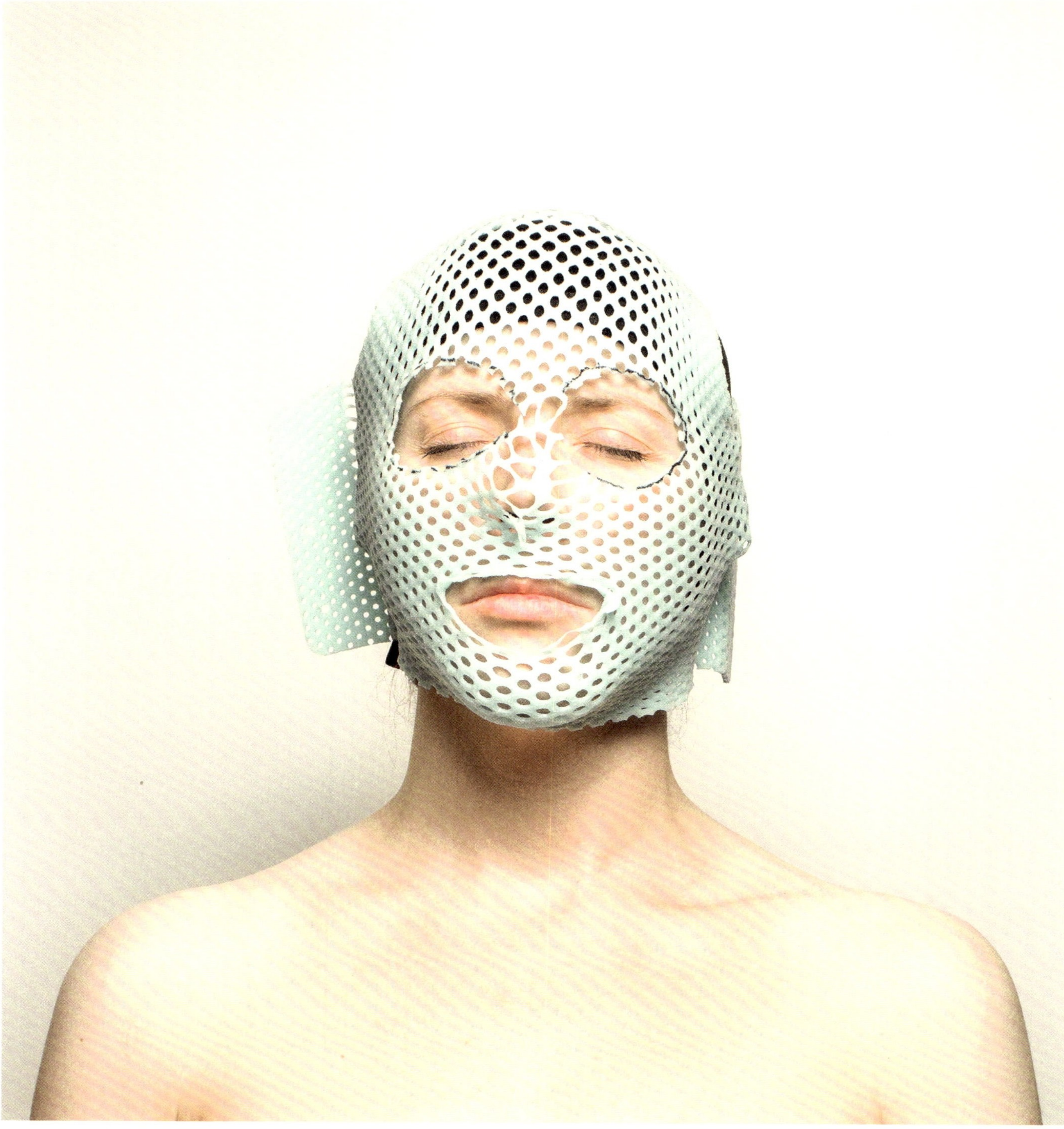

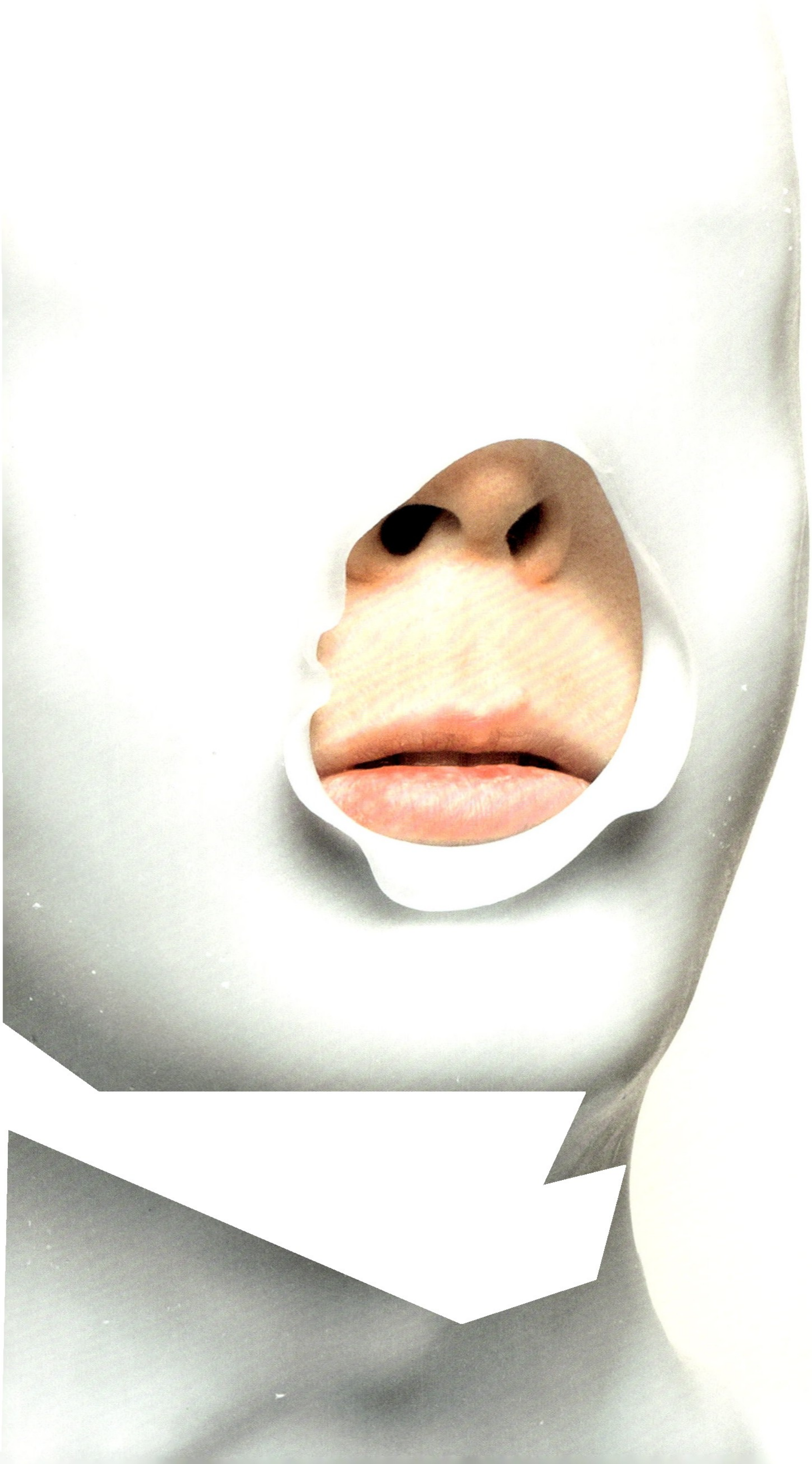

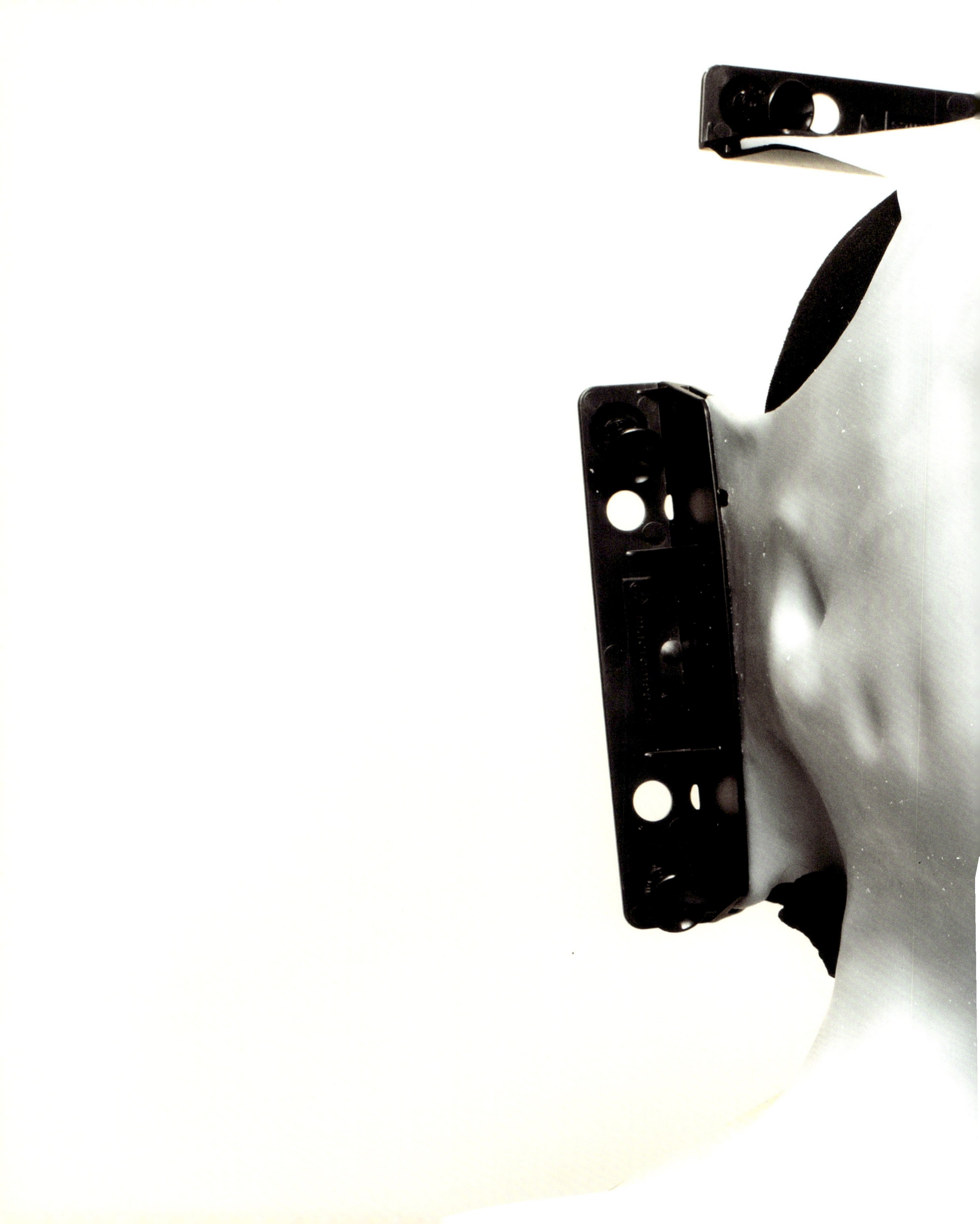

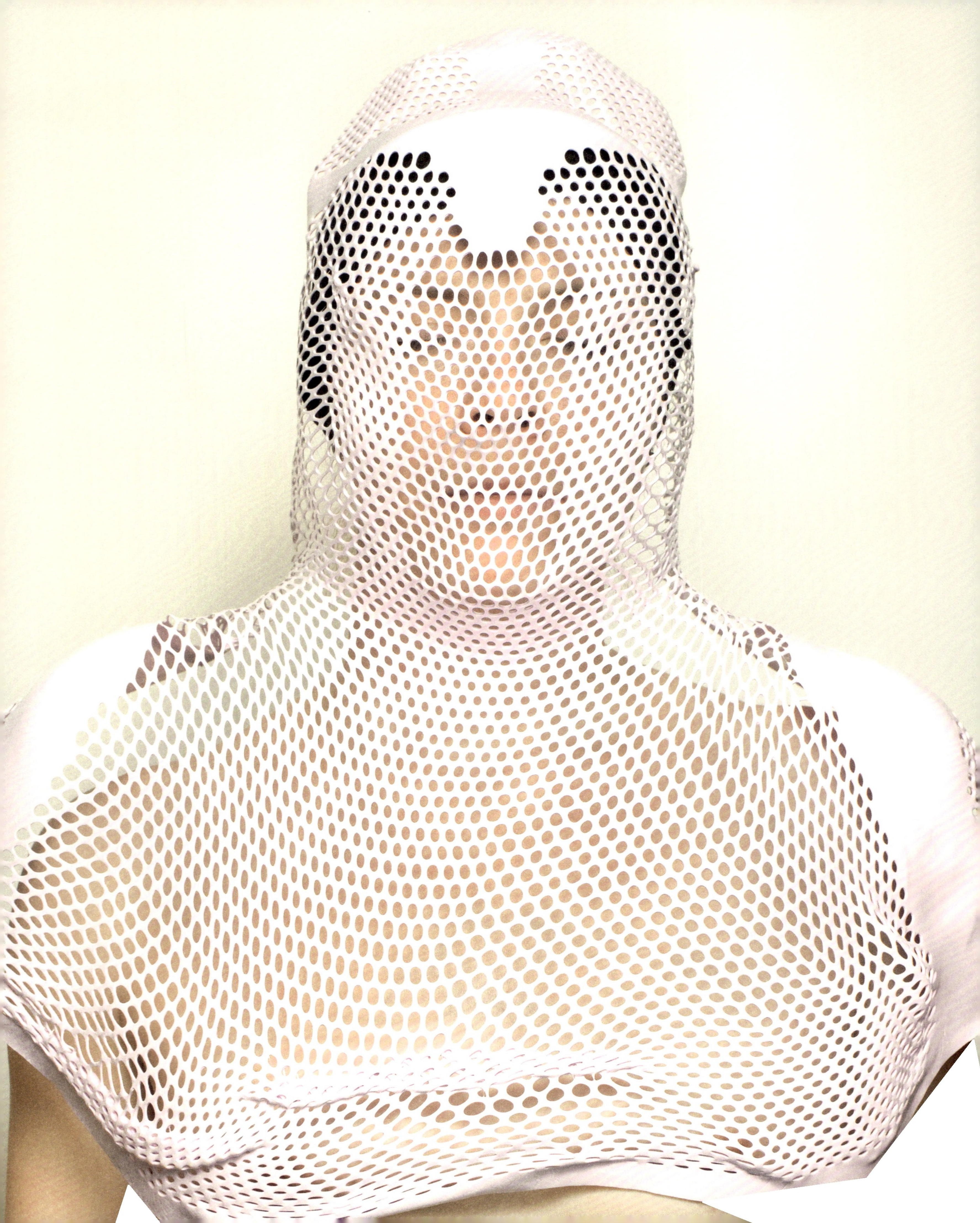

*Might help, might not. Fifty-fifty. Do you want to meet and talk about it?*

*Knowledge, treatment and hope. I have all that.*

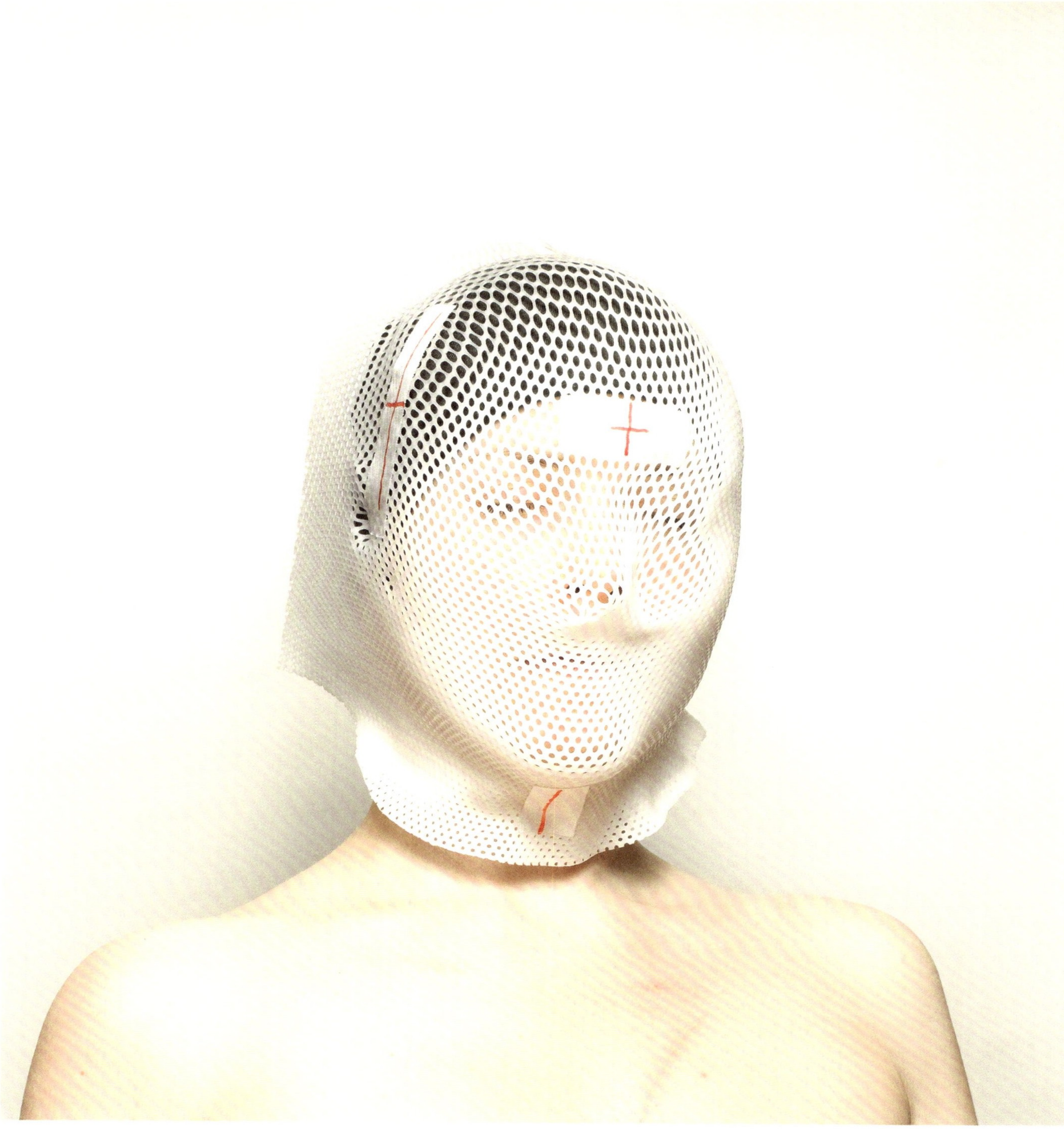

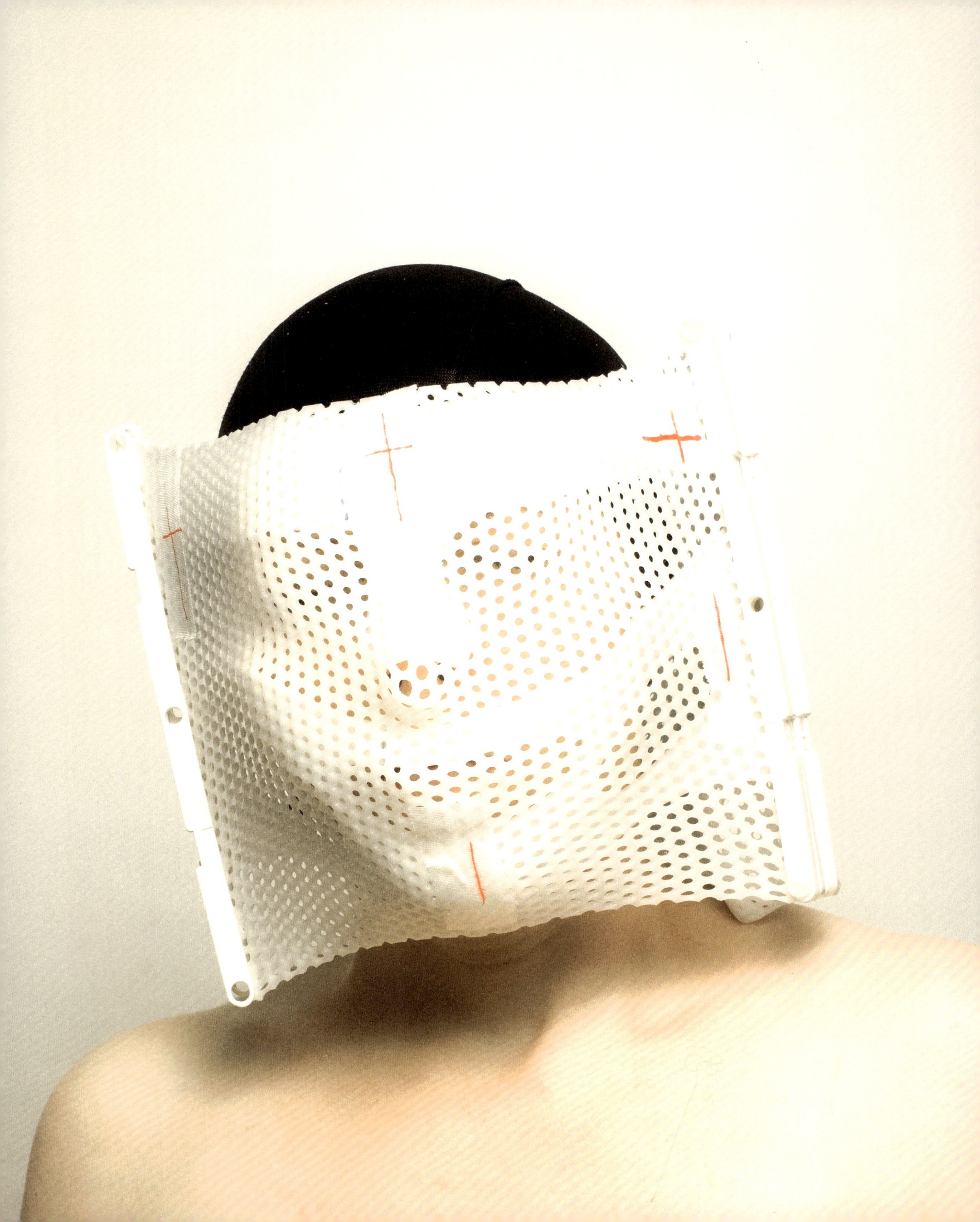

*What you want is irrelevant when it comes to me. I have no agenda.*

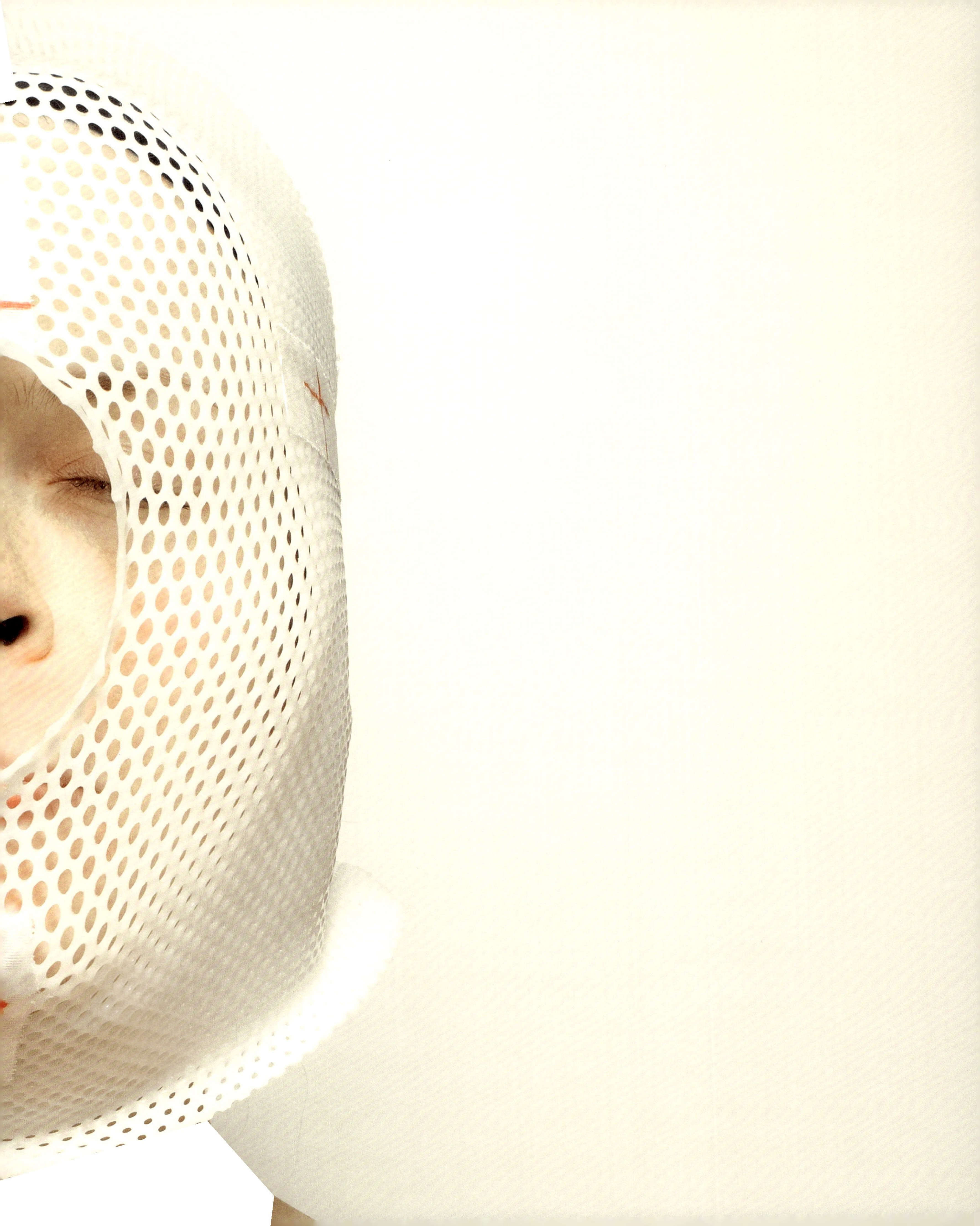

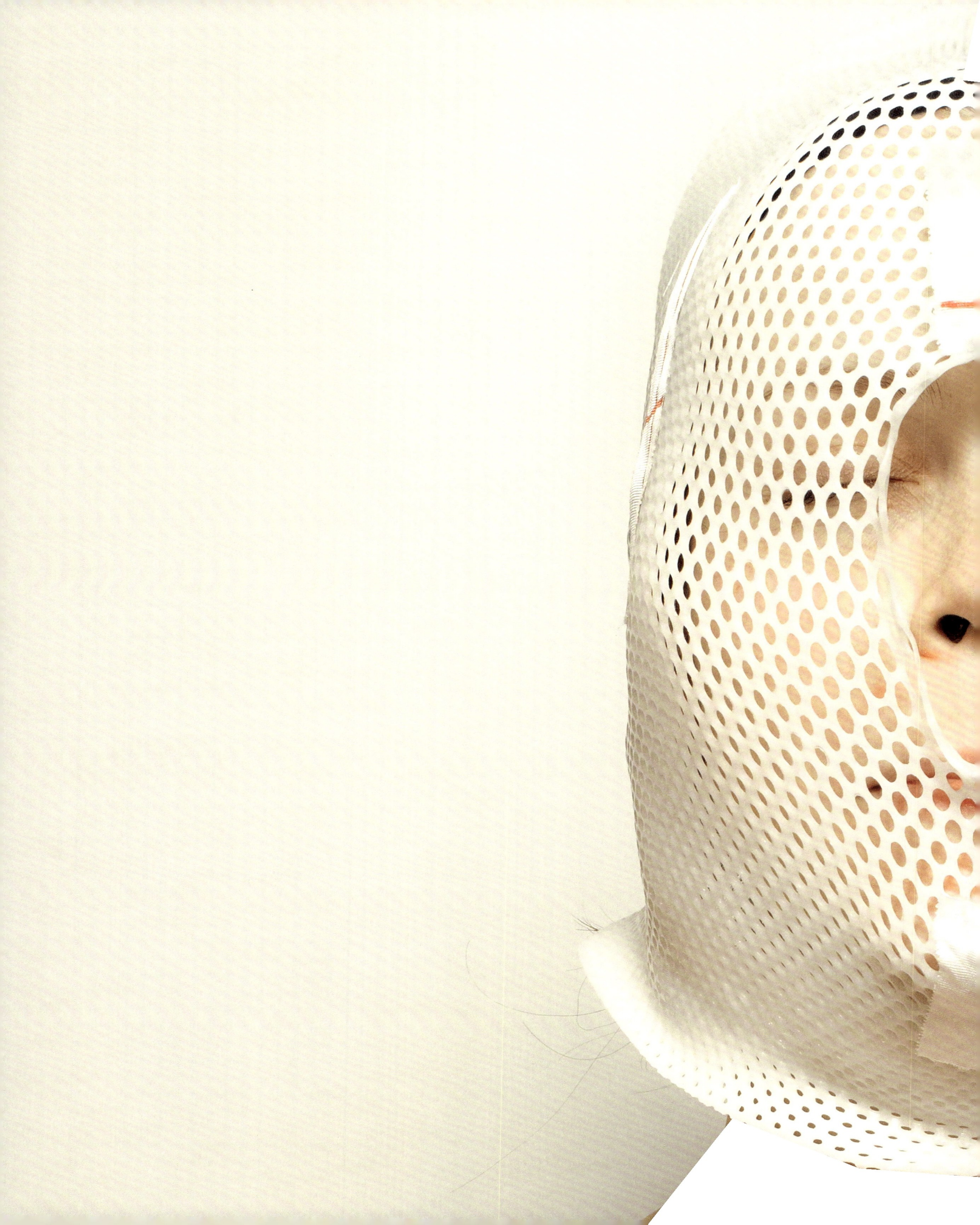

*I don't want to know you then,* I SAY.

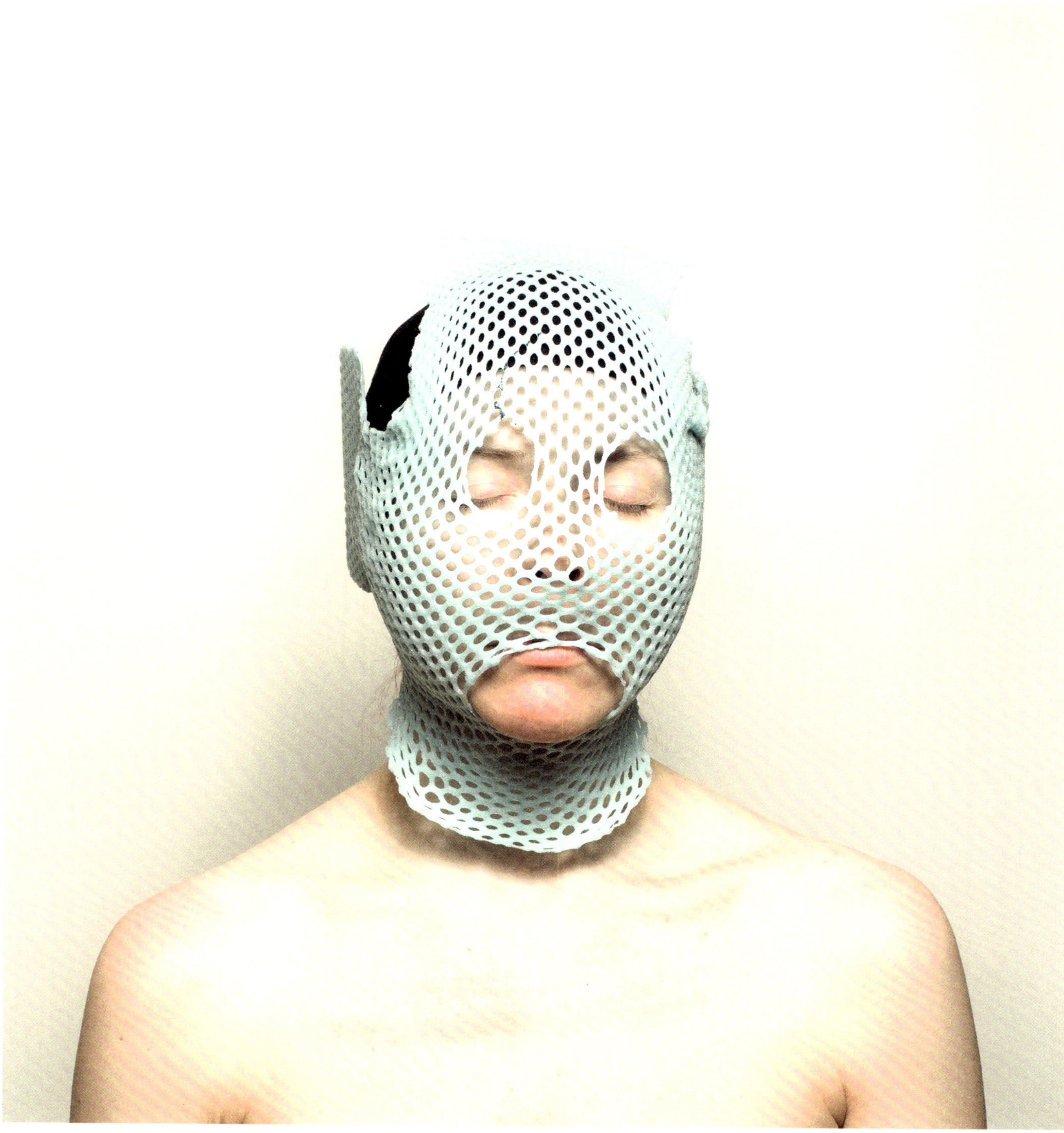

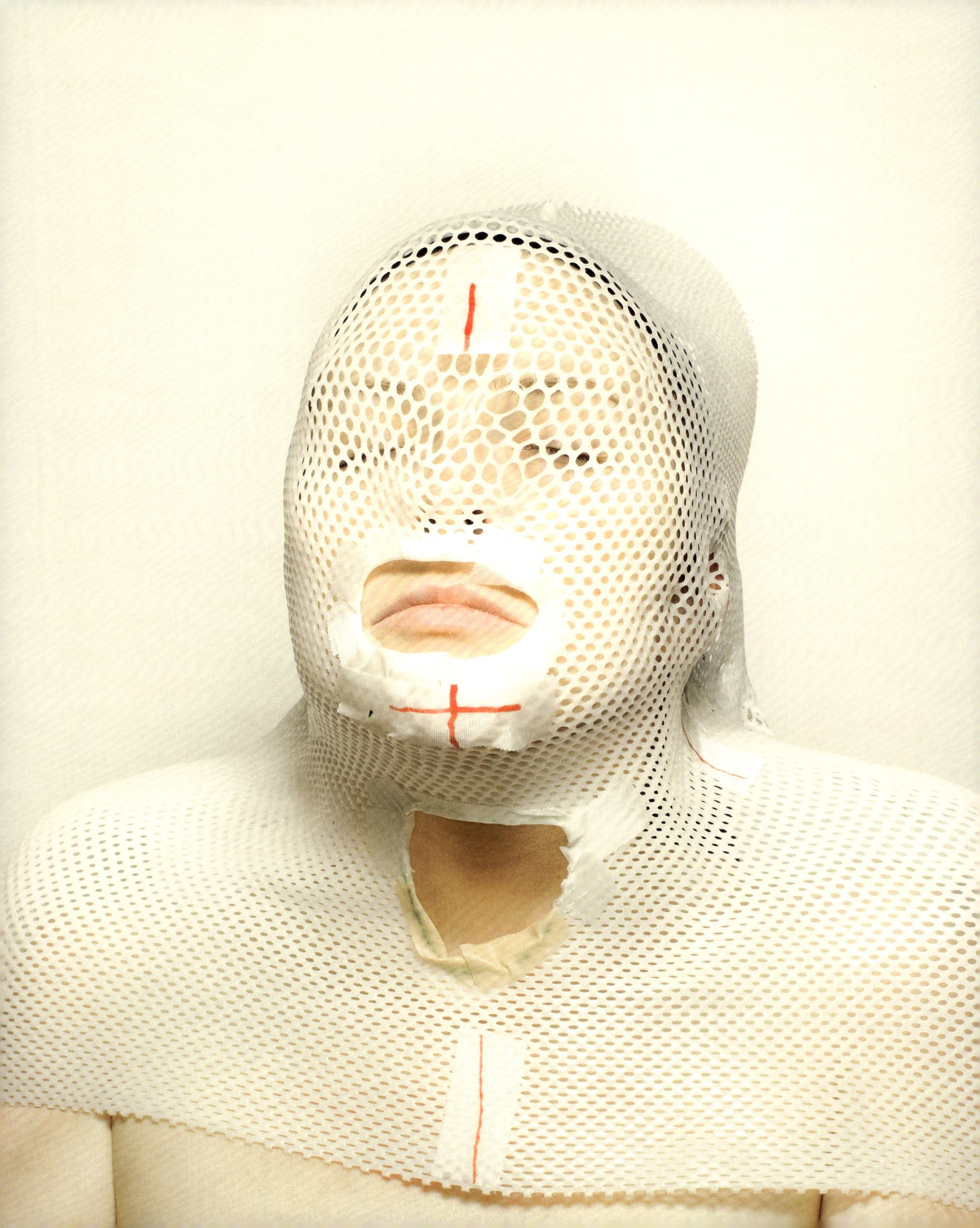

*My existence begins when you get to know me*, YOU REPLY.

*Somewhere in me, growing in secret?*

*Are you here now?*